Social Media in Clinical Practice

Bertalan Meskó

Social Media in Clinical Practice

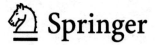 Springer

Bertalan Meskó, MD, PhD
Webicina LLC
Budapest
Hungary

ISBN 978-1-4471-4305-5   ISBN 978-1-4471-4306-2   (eBook)
DOI 10.1007/978-1-4471-4306-2
Springer London Heidelberg New York Dordrecht

Library of Congress Control Number: 2013944208

Printed on acid-free paper

Springer is part of Springer Science+Business Media (www.springer.com)

Contents

Chapter 1
Social Media Is Transforming Medicine and Healthcare

The role of the Internet in communication and information management has been becoming increasingly important for the last few years not only in medicine and healthcare, but it has been changing how we do shopping, interact with friends or organize events. The use of the Internet to search for health-related information has even become a common practice worldwide [1]. Almost everyone online is doing search queries, but actually 80 % of Internet users have looked specifically for information about health topics such as diagnosis or treatment [2].

Medical professionals are natural communicators who constantly have to communicate with patients, peers and even with information; and as social media is becoming an integral part of communication, medical professionals of the twenty-first century must acquire new skills related to digital technologies. They have to be prepared for patients asking questions about the world wide web as well.

It is now inevitable that all medical professionals regardless of their medical specialties will meet e-patients in their professional lives, therefore it is expected that doctors will need to have access to a clear guide that lets them learn skills about using the Internet for medical purposes. One of the main rationales behind writing this handbook is that while the amount of online health-related information and services is constantly growing, general population lacks of the skills to use the Internet properly for such purposes. This is also the case for medical professionals [3].

B. Meskó, *Social Media in Clinical Practice*,
DOI 10.1007/978-1-4471-4306-2_1,
© Springer-Verlag London 2013

TABLE 1.1 Main differences between the old form of Internet and social media

Old form of the Internet	Social media
Millions of users	Billions of users
Read-only content	Read-write web
Web portals and homepages	Dynamic sites (e.g. blogs, Facebook, Twitter)
One-way communication (administrators published content)	Two-way communication (users create content)
Passive – Closed	Active – Open
Static resources	Dynamic resources

Practical pieces of advice and insights into the world of digital communication with patients; online collaboration with peers; and basically the use of Internet in a medical practice are very much needed.

What Is Actually Social Media?

Throughout this book, we will refer to the Internet and mobile-based digital communication; as well as the tools of the world wide web used for interactive dialogues, forming communities and supporting user-generated content as social media. Social media was defined as "a group of Internet-based applications that build on the ideological and technological foundations of Web 2.0, and that allow the creation and exchange of user-generated content" [4]. The first term, web 2.0, referring to the changing nature of the Internet related to dynamic websites compared to the static homepages in the past was used by Tim O'Reilly in 2004 [5].

There are significant differences between the first form of the Internet and social media (Table 1.1) but the general concept of digital communication is the same. Such differences include the number of users being online; or the fact

TABLE 1.2 Comparison of web browsers

	Google Chrome	**Internet Explorer**	**Mozilla Firefox**	**Safari**
URL	http://www.google.com/chrome	http://windows.microsoft.com/en-US/internet-explorer/download-ie	http://www.mozilla.org	http://www.apple.com/safari
Cost	Free	Free with legal Windows license	Free	Free
Privacy mode (does not store browser history)	Yes	Yes	Yes	Yes
Pop-up blocking	Partial	Yes	Yes	Yes

that only administrators of websites were able to publish content while now users edit, generate and comment on content published online (e.g editing entries in Wikipedia; writing blogs or commenting on the papers in peer-reviewed journals).

Websites are accessed and browsed by using web browsers of which there are many available on the market and their development has been remarkable in the past couple of years. Choosing a web browser with the features one needs is a key step in accessing medical websites and resources [6] (Table 1.2).

Two expressions are used to refer to the medical aspects of social media, medicine 2.0 and health 2.0. Medicine 2.0 is usually associated with communication among medical professionals; while health 2.0 is more about web tools used in healthcare [7]. All stakeholders including patients, medical professionals and payers can benefit from using social media, but there are limitations and potential concerns such as privacy issues when doctors share medical cases or giving medical advice online. Although by knowing these limitations as well as the opportunities lying in the use of social media, it can become a doctor's best asset in their practice.

One of the biggest advantages of using social media for medical purposes is that it does not require any IT knowledge to leverage the power of it. Starting a new medical blog or setting up a Youtube video channel for a practice takes only a few minutes.

Studies have shown that the use of social media may be efficient for physicians (1) to keep up-to-date, (2) to share newly acquired medical knowledge with other physicians within the medical community; (3) and improve the quality of patient care [8].

Due to the constantly changing landscape of social media, its platforms and the way patients use the Internet more regularly, doctors should acquire skills needed for proper communication with their patients and peers such as assessing the quality of medical websites, using legal disclaimers in online messages or understanding the benefits and disadvantages of social media channels. As such platforms come and go, the real goal of the handbook is to provide a set of skills; concepts and a way of thinking that will assist medical professionals in analyzing the web themselves regardless of the different resources and ongoing trends.

The process during which health professionals act as gatekeepers for patients in order to identify trustworthy and credible information and services is called apomediation and is a new socio-technological term [9]. This is a crucial way to ensure patients only access quality medical information and resources online.

How Are Websites Identified?
A specific character string called uniform resource locator (URL) created in 1994 is a reference to an Internet resource (e.g. http://www.website.com).

Examples of Using Social Media in Medicine

A few real examples might shed light on how the power of social media could be used to build an online presence for a medical practice.

- A video channel on Youtube for streaming interviews and other videos.
- A Twitter account for keeping in touch with peers worldwide through short messages.
- A blog for publishing updates.
- An RSS reader to keep yourself easily up-to-date.
- Being active in a medical community site to get feedback about specific cases.
- Using medical search engines as experts to get the information we need quickly.
- Listening to podcasts while waiting in line or in a traffic jam.

Usage statistics demostrate the power and size of the most popular social networking platforms (Table 1.3).

Online Reputation

The social media era changed the way patients find medical professionals or healthcare institutions as they check their online presence first and what they find there will be decisive. As we do more and more regular tasks on the web, our online profile is now a part of how patients choose us. Therefore establishing a well-designed and controlled profile in the Internet has benefits.

My own profile includes:

- A LinkedIn account with CV and other detailed pieces of information of my professional career (http://www.linkedin.com/in/bertalanmesko).
- A Twitter account that connects me to peers worldwide with its own customized design (https://twitter.com/Berci) (Fig. 1.1).

TABLE 1.3 Comparison of the most popular social networking platforms

Name of the social networking site (URL)	Description	Number of registered users as of 2013 [10]
Twitter (http://twitter.com)	Microblogging	500 million
Facebook (http://facebook.com)	Community site	One billion
Youtube (http://youtube.com)	Video sharing site	cc. 800 million
Google+ (http://plus.google.com)	Community site	400 million
Flickr (http://www.flickr.com)	Photo sharing site	32 million

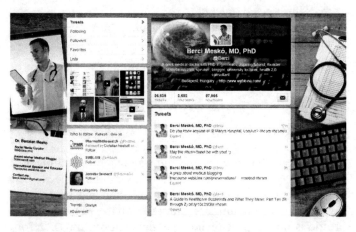

FIGURE 1.1 My Twitter profile

- A blog focusing on my professional activities and projects (http://www.scienceroll.com).
- A website serving as a hub for all my online channels (http://medicalfuturist.com/).

The best way to control what kind of information others will find about us online is to control it ourselves by providing quality content and/or creating well-designed profiles in professional community sites (Fig. 1.2).

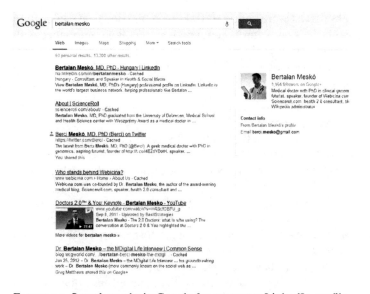

FIGURE 1.2 Search results in Google for my name: LinkedIn profile, own medical blog, own Twitter channel, own company, video and written interviews (Google and the Google logo are registered trademarks of Google Inc., used with permission)

Assessing the Quality of Medical Websites and Platforms

As patients have questions about the Internet such as where they can find blogs or community sites about their own condition during a regular doctor visit, medical professionals have to learn assess the quality of medical websites and other platforms online. Moreover, in the modern Internet era, medical professionals should also be able to "prescribe information" for their patients in an evidence-based manner.

The so-called "Information therapy" could improve patient knowledge, decision making, and communication, as the availability of online health information does not ensure improved knowledge or better health decisions by patients are associated to the access to information. Patients received such prescribed information therapy from their primary care physicians were reported to have a high level of satisfaction with their care, improved health status, and compliance with prescriptions [11].

The assessment of the quality of medical websites and platforms requires the analysis of the following parameters:

- Contact information of the authors (e.g. e-mail address, phone number).
- The blog has a title, optionally a sub-title and a description of the mission of the site.
- Description of the author or authors with work address and affiliation.
- Archives represent a long-time commitment to providing information online but does not ensure high quality.
- The availability of a properly formatted RSS feed and numerous feed readers is a good sign.
- Privacy policy is a legal document that describes the ways the website or platform owners gather, use, disclose and manage a customer or reader's data.
- A disclaimer is a statement intended to specify the scope of the site as well as obligations that may be exercised by parties in a legally recognized relationship. A medical disclaimer should be made visible on all websites dealing with medical information highlighting that the information provided on the website is intended only for educational purposes, not medical ones.
- Statements, facts and data should be referenced in the entries or articles on the website. The source of the images, figures and photos should always be highlighted.
- The information on the website must comply with the Health Insurance Portability and Accountability Act (HIPAA), a law enacted in the US that protects health insurance coverage for workers and their families when they change or lose their jobs; and also addresses the security and privacy of health data [12].
- Certifications make the assessment easier. The Health On the Net Foundation (HONcode) is a not-for-profit organization founded in 1995 under the auspices of the Geneva Ministry of Health in order to supervise the quality of medical websites and blogs [13]. Webicina (http://www.webicina.com)

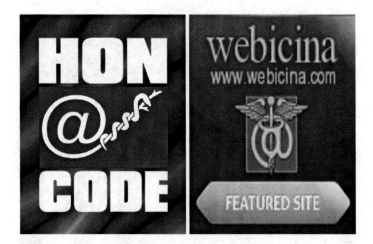

FIGURE 1.3 The HONcode and Webicina banners

is an online service that curates medical websites and social media resources [14] (Fig. 1.3).

In most cases, websites or online platforms do not provide all of these, therefore the decision is generally not easy. The analysis of more and more websites and social media platforms gives you confidence and experience which are the key elements in the process of assessment (Figs. 1.4 and 1.5).

Self-Test

1. What is social media?
   Web and mobile-based digital communication, and the tools of the world wide web used for interactive dialogues, forming communities and supporting user-generated content.
2. What is the most prominent difference between the old form of web and social media?
   Social media is referring to the read-write web in which users can edit content.
3. What is the process of health professionals acting as gatekeepers for patients in order to identify trustworthy and credible information and services called?
   Apomediation.

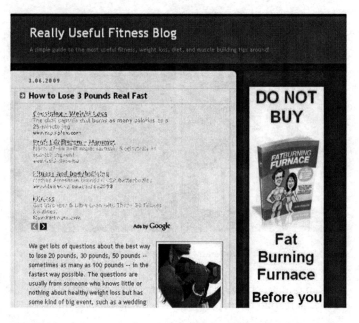

FIGURE 1.4 An example for a low quality website. Subtitle is missing, advertisements are in the sidebar and between entries, no references included in the entries, no source of image is highlighted, author information, site description, archives, privacy policy and disclaimer are not available

Next Steps

1. Do a search online for your name and see what people find about you.
2. Write a plan what kind of information you would like others to find about you.
3. See what social networking sites you have already been using [10].
4. Check your profiles for personal and professional content (these should be separated).
5. Find colleagues in those networks and see what they share.
6. Choose those networks that seem to be useful for your purposes.

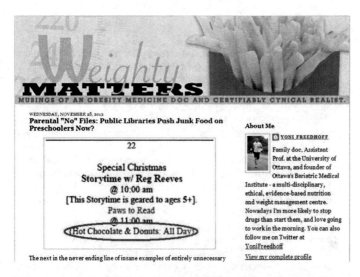

FIGURE 1.5 An example for a high quality website. Custom design, blog title and subtitle as well as a short description are available on the main page. Author information and contact details are shown. Over 1,500 RSS readers and references in the articles ensure high quality

Key Points
- There are no differences regarding the general concept between social media and the old form of the world wide web.
- Digital communication is playing an immense role in medicine and healthcare.
- E-patients are leading the movement and medical professionals should acquire skills in digital literacy.
- Using specific quality features, the value of medical websites can be assessed, though it requires practice.

References

1. AlGhamdi KM, Moussa NA. Internet use by the public to search for health-related information. Int J Med Inform. 2012;81(6):363–73.
2. Pew Internet: the social life of health information. 2011. http://pewinternet.org/Reports/2011/Social-Life-of-Health-Info/Summary-of-Findings.aspx. Accessed 8 Aug 2012.
3. Van Deursen AJAM, Van Dijk JAGM. Internet skills performance tests: are people ready for ehealth? J Med Internet Res. 2011; 13(2):e35.
4. Kaplan AM, Haenlein M. Users of the world, unite! The challenges and opportunities of Social Media. Bus Horiz. 2010;53(1):59–68.
5. http://www.paulgraham.com/web20.html. Accessed 19 Mar 2013.
6. http://en.wikipedia.org/wiki/Comparison_of_web_browsers. Accessed 24 Jan 2013.
7. Van De Belt TH, et al. Definition of Health 2.0 and Medicine 2.0: a systematic review. J Med Internet Res. 2010;12(2):e18.
8. McGowan B, et al. Understanding the factors that influence the adoption and meaningful use of social media by physicians to share medical information. J Med Internet Res. 2012;14(5):e117.
9. Eysenbach G. Medicine 2.0: social networking, collaboration, participation, apomediation, and openness. J Med Internet Res. 2008; 10(3):Art e22.
10. http://en.wikipedia.org/wiki/List_of_social_networking_websites. Accessed 19 Mar 2013.
11. Keene N, et al. Preliminary benefits of information therapy. J Prim Care Community Health. 2011;2(1):45–8.
12. http://www.hhs.gov/ocr/privacy/index.html. Accessed 17 Dec 2012.
13. http://www.hon.ch/HONcode/Conduct.html. Accessed 17 Dec 2012.
14. http://www.webicina.com/. Accessed 17 Dec 2012.

Chapter 2
Using Medical Search Engines with a Special Focus on Google

There are billions of pages on the World Wide Web and search engines help us find the information we are looking for. Having so many pages with a huge amount of information online is the biggest advantage and disadvantage of the Internet at the same time. Instead of manually browsing the websites, search engines point us to the pages that contain the key words we are looking for.

How Do Search Engines Work?

Search engines use robots (also known as spiders or crawlers) which are programs that can automatically follow hyperlinks from one document to another one sending information about new sites back to its main repository to be indexed. Due to the dynamic nature of many websites, robots keep an index of words they find and the place where they find them; and do this indexing process regularly even on websites that had previously been catalogued. It means new websites or new content on known websites have to be indexed first in order to become accessible through search engines.

The Short History of Search Engines

It is not surprising using e-mails and search engines are the two most common practices online [1]. Due to this fact, the first widely adopted search engine was launched back in 1995

B. Meskó, *Social Media in Clinical Practice*,
DOI 10.1007/978-1-4471-4306-2_2,
© Springer-Verlag London 2013

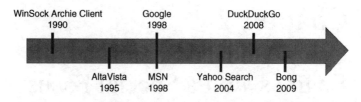

FIGURE 2.1 Timeline of the appearance of search engines

under the name AltaVista (http://www.altavista.com/) and other search engines were created soon after that (Fig. 2.1). As of 2013, the most popular search engines globally are Google (https://www.google.com/), Bing (http://www.bing.com/), Yahoo (http://www.yahoo.com/), Ask (http://ask.com/) and AOL (http://www.aol.com/) [2].

Out of these search engines, Google seemed to attract the most people (over one billion users as of 2012) [3]. It was founded by Larry Page and Sergey Brin on September 4, 1998 while they attended Stanford University. The name Google originates from a misspelling of the word "googol" accounting for the number one followed by one hundred zeros.

The Basics of Searching Online

On the main page, search queries can be inserted into the box and search results can be obtained by clicking on the Google Search button. A faster alternative is clicking on the "I'm Feeling Lucky" button which immediately takes the user to the first entry of the search results assuming that one is the best possible resource (Fig. 2.2.).

A typical page of search results features a sidebar on the left or on the top showing additional search functions such as searching only for images, maps, videos or news, among others. The number of search results and the time needed to come up with those are listed below the search box that contains the search query. For each search results, the title of the website, the URL and a short description of that particular website are shown (Fig. 2.3).

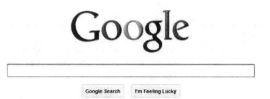

FIGURE 2.2 The main page of Google.com (Google and the Google logo are registered trademarks of Google Inc., used with permission)

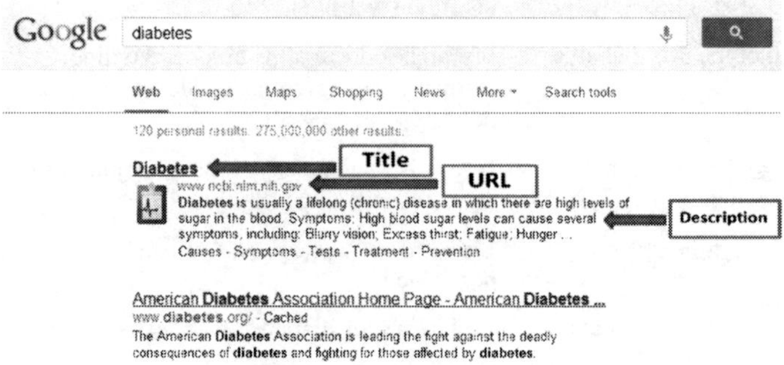

FIGURE 2.3 A search query on "diabetes" on Google.com (Google and the Google logo are registered trademarks of Google Inc., used with permission)

The order of the search results is determined based on the so-called page rank of the websites. Each website that is indexed by the robots of Google gets a score ranging from 1 to 10. This is called pagerank; and the more and better connections the website has with other websites, the higher the pagerank is making it appear in the search results.

There are numerous tricks and operators that can facilitate the use of search engines such as removing words from the query or searching only on a specific website; or for a specific filetype. Examples are summarized in Table 2.1.

In cases when rules do not permit the use of search engines that track user information DuckDuckGo

TABLE 2.1 Search operators in Google.com

Search query	What it does
diabetes OR allergy	Search for websites containing either of the words, otherwise it would typically show sites that contain both
diabetes AND allergy	Search for websites that contain both words
-diabetes	It shows websites that do not contain the search term
site:www.example.com diabetes	It searches for the keyword on only the identified website
filetype:doc diabetes	It searches documents uploaded online featuring the search term. File type can be pdf or ppt, among others
"diabetes treatment options"	It searches for exactly this expression in this word order
5 kg in pound	Unit and money conversions can be performed
inurl:WHO diabetes	It searches for diabetes in all web pages that have "WHO" in their URLs
intitle:diabetes	It searches for diabetes in the titles of web pages and documents instead of the body of the text

(http://www.duckduckgo.com) serves as an alternative being a search engine that emphasizes privacy and does not record user information therefore all users receive the same search results for a given search query.

What Is Search Engine Optimization (SEO)?

SEO is a common term used all around the web, and it refers to the process of improving the visibility of a website in search engines by inserting the right key words in the right places in the content.

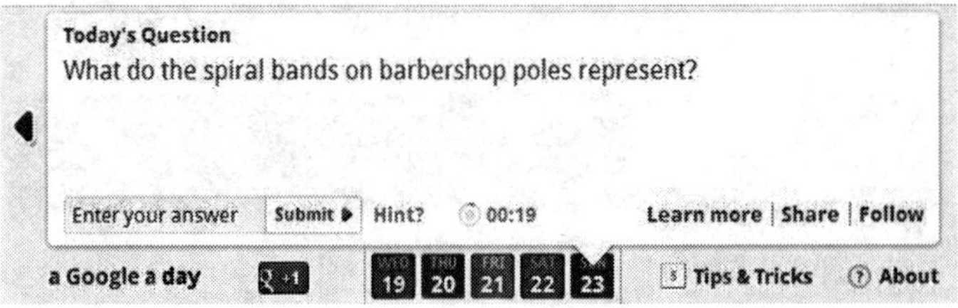

Today's Question
What do the spiral bands on barbershop poles represent?

Enter your answer   Submit ▶   Hint?   ⊙ 00:19   Learn more | Share | Follow

a Google a day   ☒ +1   19 20 21 22 23   ⑤ Tips & Tricks   ⑦ About

FIGURE 2.4 A Google A Day provides daily search tasks with solutions (Google and the Google logo are registered trademarks of Google Inc., used with permission)

How to Get Better at Searching Online?

A list of suggestions and tips that can help obtain better search results:

- Be as precise as possible.
- Focus only on the keywords of your query, the rarest words in the sentence or question.
- Fasten searches by using the right operators (e.g. AND, OR, intitle, author, etc.).
- Narrow your search results in more steps, first results do not necessarily lead to the information you are looking for.
- Think as if you published the information you are looking for and what kind of keywords you would have been using.

If you are looking for PDF documents that mention diabetes in their title but do not contain the word treatment in their content, the best way to do so is to search for "filetype:PDF intitle:diabetes –treatment" which will show only relevant results. This example underscores the importance of using different search operators at once with strategy.

An ideal strategy for getting better at online searches is practising more by using the right queries, keywords and operators in order to save time and effort every day. Methods for structured learning include "A Google A Day" (http://www.agoogleaday.com) that provides questions and tasks related to special search queries every day by showing the solution in the form of specific search queries and keywords as well (Fig. 2.4).

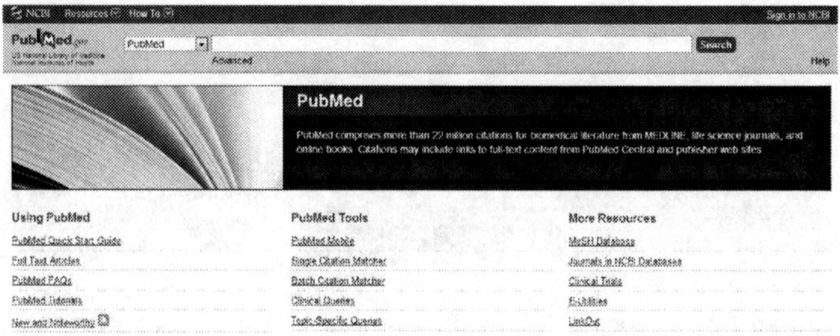

FIGURE 2.5 The main page of http://www.Pubmed.com

Search Engines in Medicine and Research

Pubmed.com

Certain search engines index the whole world wide web while others focus on topics and sub-topics such as medicine and research. The most prominent example is Pubmed.com which was launched by The United States National Library of Medicine at the National Institutes of Health in 1996 and includes over 22 million citations serving as a repository of the biomedical literature [4] (Fig. 2.5).

Instead of searching for a specific field of interest or research topic regularly, making these search queries automatic facilitates our work flow for which there are basically two methods.

Registering a free account on Pubmed.com and clicking on "Save Search" below a search query sets up e-mail alerts to receive the latest publications focusing on these keywords automatically (Figs. 2.6, 2.7, and 2.8).

The second method includes doing searches for keywords and clicking on the RSS button below it which makes it possible to create RSS feeds out of the search query which can be added to RSS readers therefore all the upcoming papers focusing on our field of interest will be syndicated to our RSS reader (Fig. 2.9).

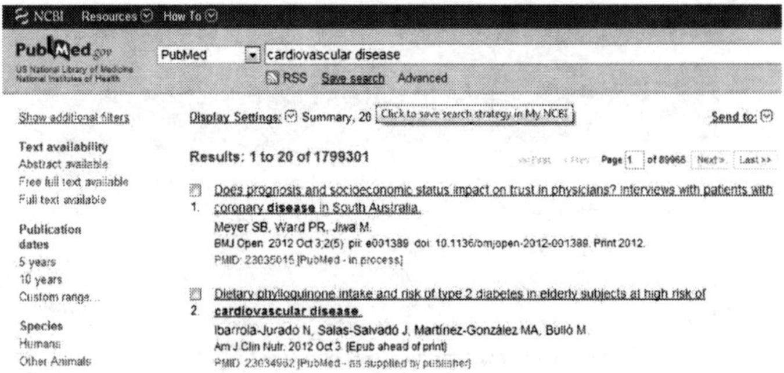

FIGURE 2.6 A common search results page on Pubmed.com. Filtering options can be found in the left sidebar

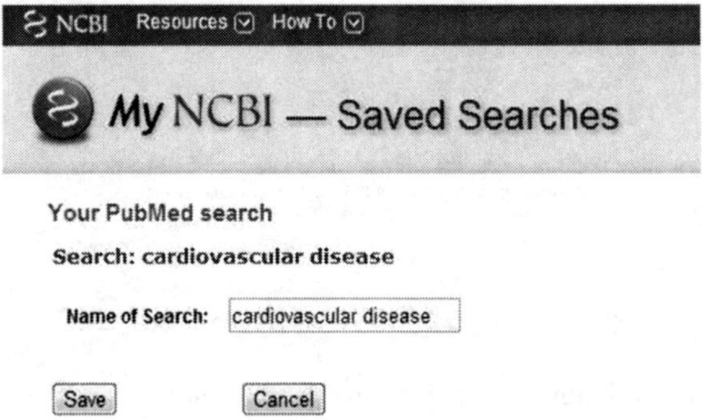

FIGURE 2.7 Dashboard after clicking on "Save search" on Pubmed. com

Third-Party Pubmed Tools

As the US National Library of Medicine released the application programming interface (API) through which other services and online platforms can access the database, third-party Pubmed tools were introduced such as GoPubmed (http://www.gopubmed.org), BibliMed (http:// www.biblimed.com) or Pubget (http://pubget.com). These

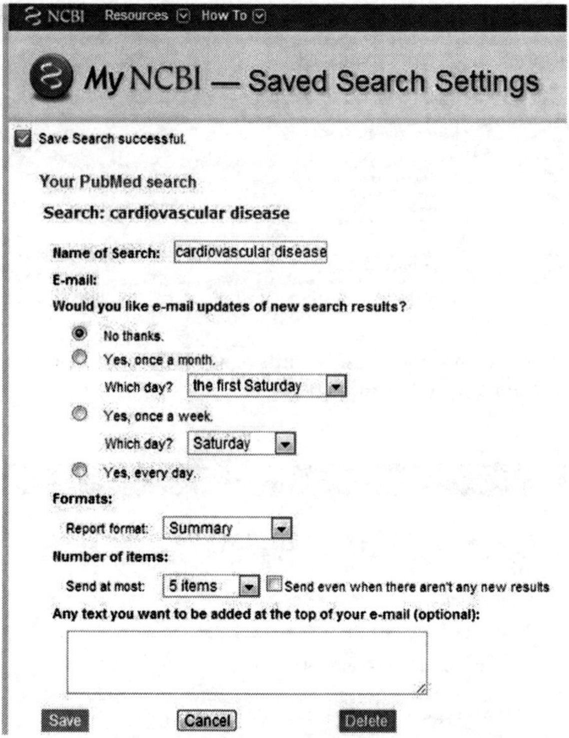

FIGURE 2.8 Settings using the "Save search" button

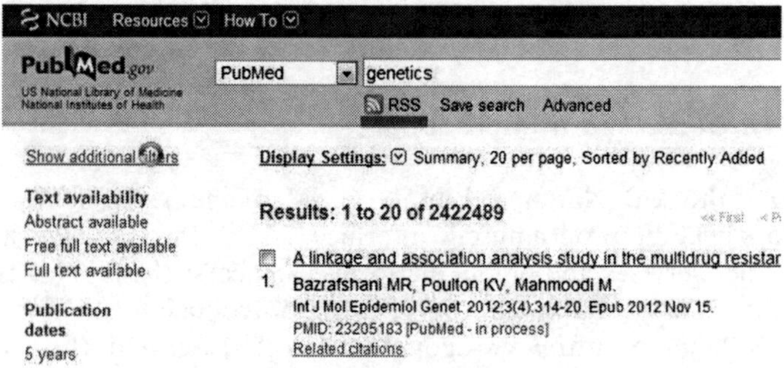

FIGURE 2.9 The RSS button is below the search box on Pubmed.com

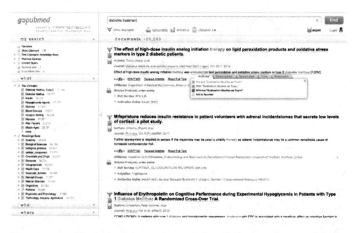

FIGURE 2.10 The page of search results on Gopubmed.com with the additional filtering options in the left sidebar. A third-party Pubmed tool mixes the database of NCBI and the technological advantages of other search engines

are knowledge-based search engines specifically designed to search for biomedical texts significantly faster than Pubmed (Fig. 2.10).

These make it possible to narrow search results by different identifiers including authors, sub-topics or publication date in an easy-to-use interface.

Google Scholar

Launched in 2004, Google Scholar (http://scholar.google.com) is a search engine that indexes the full text of scholarly literature, most peer reviewed journals, scholarly books and other non-peer reviewed journals. Google Scholar allows users to search for digital or physical copies of articles, technical reports, preprints, theses, books, and patents (Fig. 2.11).

It works similarly to other search engines but there are several tools for customization of the search results such as

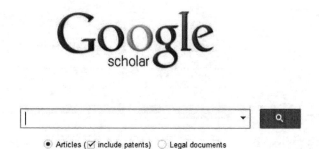

● Articles (☑ include patents) ○ Legal documents

FIGURE 2.11 The search box on Google Scholar. Basic settings include searching in patents as well besides research articles (Google and the Google logo are registered trademarks of Google Inc., used with permission)

filtering by date, relevance or document type. It also shows how many times a paper were cited by other papers or whether there are other versions available of a particular article (Fig. 2.12).

Similarly to the search engine of Google, search operators can be used in Google Scholar as well in order to make more customized search queries (Table 2.2).

In order to receive automatic updates of the newest additions focusing on a specific search query, alerts can be set up by using the "Create alert" function in the bottom left corner. By providing a valid e-mail address, updates will be sent from time to time (Fig. 2.13).

WolframAlpha

Wolfram Alpha (http://www.wolframalpha.com) developed by Wolfram Research is an online search engine that answers factual queries by computing the answer from structured data. Numerous medical databases have been uploaded in different fields of medicine from public health to laboratory results [5]. Instead of providing a list of relevant websites and articles, WolframAlpha aims at giving the final answer right away.

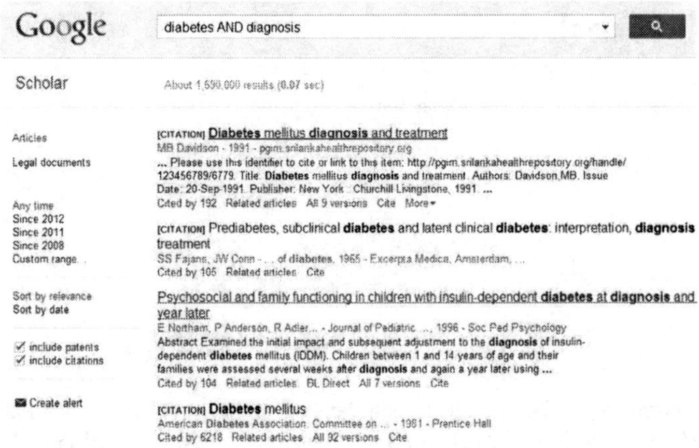

FIGURE 2.12 The search results' page on Google Scholar. Filtering options are shown in the left sidebar and citations of each paper can be accessed below the results (Google and the Google logo are registered trademarks of Google Inc., used with permission)

TABLE 2.2 Additional search operators that could be used in Google Scholar as well

Search operator	What it does
+word	Adds a word to the search
-word	Removes a word from the search
crohn OR diabetes	Searches for articles containing either of the words
author:Brown	Searches for authors named Brown
intitle:diabetes	Searches for articles that feature the word diabetes in their titles

Examples of medical search queries on WolframAlpha (with the exact search query):

- compute estimated risk of heart disease ("heart disease risk 50 year-old male")
- get gender and age-specific information about a test result ("creatinine = 0.9 mg/dL, adult male")

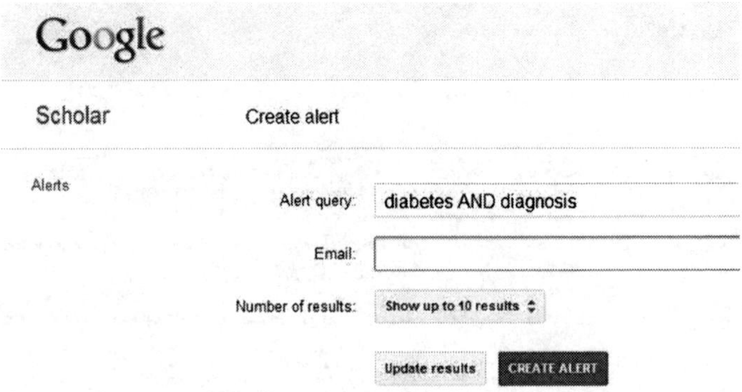

FIGURE 2.13 E-mail alerts can be set up using Google Scholar (Google and the Google logo are registered trademarks of Google Inc., used with permission)

- compute various body statistics based on height, weight, etc. ("BMI 5′10″, 165 lb")
- get an overview of health care costs in a country ("Canada healthcare expenditures")

Self-Test

1. Which search engine should I use?
   There are minor differences between the most popular search engines, give the top three a try and you will be able to choose. Speed and safety can be the major features.
2. How can I search for PDF documents in diabetes?
   Use the relevant operators such as "filetype:pdf diabetes".
3. How can I receive updates in my academic field of interest automatically?
   Both Google Scholar and Pubmed offer e-mail alerts or RSS feeds.

Next Steps

1. Do a couple of search queries for your name, workplace and field of interests.
2. Do the same search queries in the three major search engines (Google, Bing, Yahoo).
3. See what kind of search operators you could use [6].
4. Pratice your skills for a few days or weeks on "A Google a Day".

Key Points
- Search engines help find the content, websites or pieces of information you need.
- Focus on keywords and use the search query operators.
- Set up automatic alerts on Pubmed in order to receive the latest updates in a field of interest.
- Use Google Scholar and Pubmed together for the best results in academic search.
- WolframAlpha provides excellent computational solutions in medicine and healthcare.

References

1. Pew Internet: the social life of health information. 2011. http://pewinternet.org/Reports/2011/Social-Life-of-Health-Info/Summary-of-Findings.aspx. Accessed 8 Aug 2012.
2. Top 15 Most Popular Search Engines. http://www.ebizmba.com/articles/search-engines
3. Google's new record, 1 billion visitors in May. http://itsalltech.com/2011/06/22/googles-new-record-1-billion-visitors-in-may/. Accessed 4 Sept 2012.
4. http://en.wikipedia.org/wiki/PubMed. Accessed 28 Jan 2013.
5. http://www.wolframalpha.com/examples/HealthAndMedicine.html. Accessed 24 Jan 2013.
6. http://www.googleguide.com/advanced_operators.html. Accessed 20 Mar 2013.

Chapter 3
Being Up-to-Date in Medicine

Being up-to-date is crucial in medicine as the amount of information available in any specialties is skyrocketing. This information pollution is causing a major and constantly growing challenge for medical professionals as well.

The old methods of sitting in the library checking a few papers every week is not a sustainable solution any more. Publishing in the medical literature and the search for peer-reviewed papers now require the use of the Internet, therefore we can go online for keeping ourselves up-to-date. The world wide web can only facilitate our workflow if the right tools are used. But instead of browsing the web and looking for new content relevant to our needs, information should come to us in a structured, controlled and efficient way.

In this chapter, methods for letting the information come to us as well as methods for following the literature, our citations or websites mentioning our work are presented.

Using RSS

RSS which was used to be an abbreviation for RDF Site Summary, then Rich Site Summary, now Really Simple Syndication can be described as a family of web feed formats for delivering regularly updated web content such as blogs, news sites, audio and video channels in a standardized way. An RSS document that was first introduced in 1995 (feed or

B. Meskó, *Social Media in Clinical Practice*,   27
DOI 10.1007/978-1-4471-4306-2_3,
© Springer-Verlag London 2013

FIGURE 3.1 The most commonly used icon of RSS

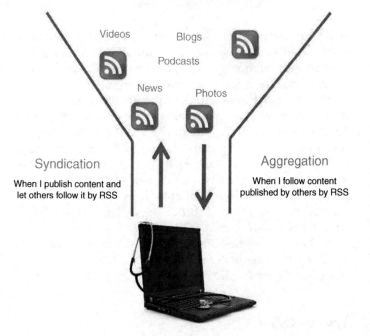

FIGURE 3.2 Schematic view of the advantages of using RSS

channel) includes text, date of publishing and information on authorship [1] (Fig. 3.1).

Author or publishers of dynamic content such as blogs or news sites can syndicate their content automatically and readers can aggregate these in a very simple way without checking for new content on each website [2] (Fig. 3.2).

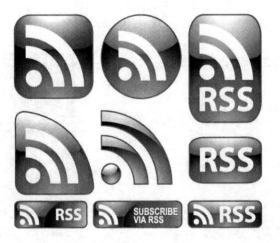

FIGURE 3.3 Different icons of RSS

Web-based, desktop-based or mobile device-based softwares called an "RSS reader", "feed reader", or "RSS aggregator" can read RSS feeds. Readers can subscribe to the feeds of different websites and the new content of all the channels the user subscribed to will be updated automatically in the RSS reader. As soon as the new content is available in those channels, it appears immediately in the RSS reader therefore there is no need to manually check the news any more but we let the information come to us and by checking only one place (our RSS reader), all the information we need are delivered (Fig. 3.3).

How to Subscribe to an RSS Feed?

Web-based tools make it possible to read RSS channels one is subscribed to on any computers or mobile devices as all the settings are stored online. Examples include Feedly (http://www.feedly.com) which is a widely used RSS reader. It works across most web browsers such as Chrome, Firefox and Safari, as well as mobile devices running IOS and Android. Let's subscribe to the RSS feed of a medical journal.

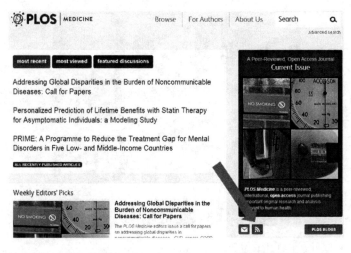

FIGURE 3.4 The RSS icon on the main page of PLoS Medicine

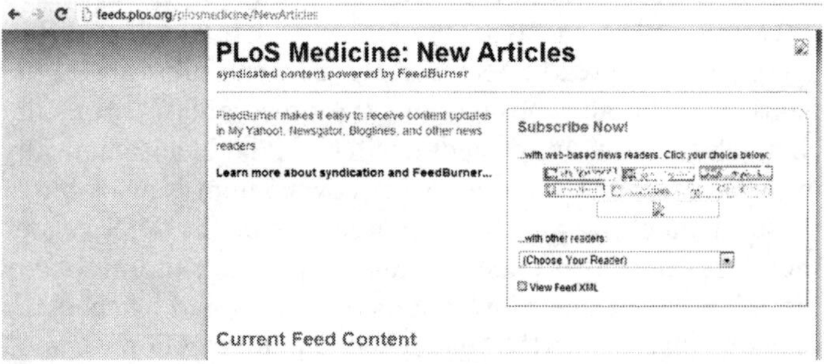

FIGURE 3.5 Clicking on the RSS icon leads users to this page of the RSS feed

Step 1: Go to the website of your preferred journal (in this case PLoS Medicine is the example we use - http://www.plosmedicine.org/) (Fig. 3.4).

Step 2: Look for the common symbol of RSS feeds (indicated by a red arrow in Fig. 3.4) and click on that.

Step 3: After being redirected to a new page, copy the URL above (Fig. 3.5).

Step 4: Open Feedly, click on "Add Content" and insert the URL of that RSS feed into the search box. It will let

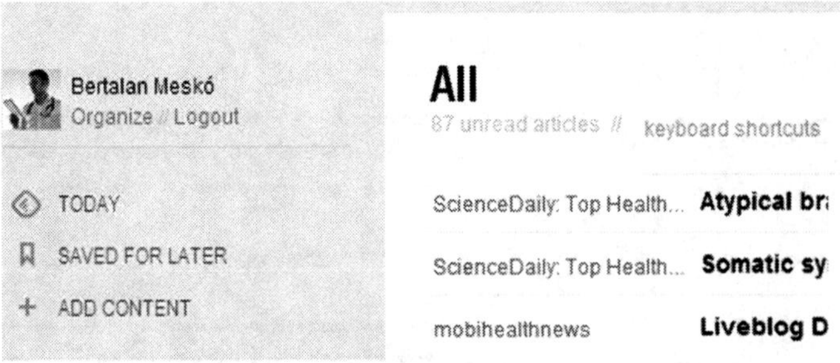

FIGURE 3.6 The main page of Feedly where RSS feeds can be inserted

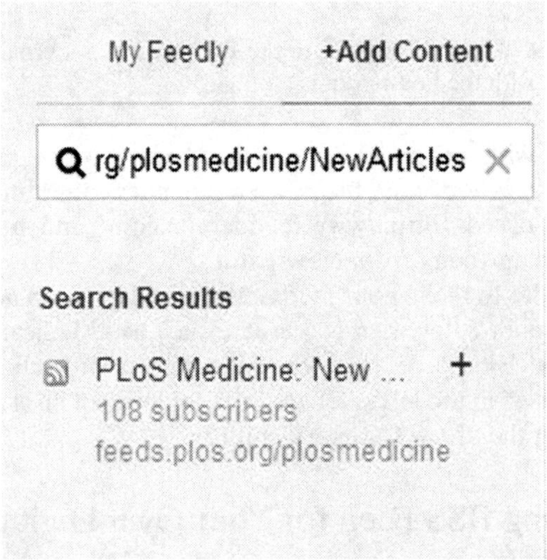

FIGURE 3.7 Searching for a website, topic or specific RSS feed lets users add the content to the database on Feedly with the plus sign

you add it to your database with the plus sign. Otherwise, based on your preferences, Feedly also adds any RSS feeds to your database only by clicking on the RSS icon in a web browser (Figs. 3.6 and 3.7).

You just subscribed to the RSS feed of a medical journal (Fig. 3.8). The same process works with blogs, news sites and any other dynamic platforms with active RSS channels as

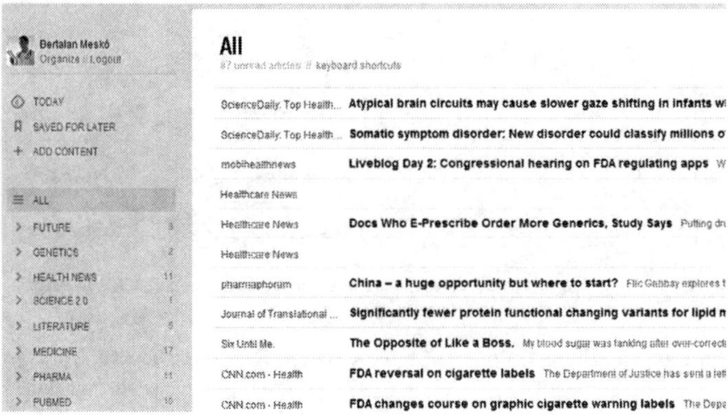

FIGURE 3.8 After subscribing to the RSS feed of a journal leads to this page with the latest entries

well as with other RSS readers whether those are web- (http://my.yahoo.com/, http://www.bloglines.com/), mobile or desktop-based (http://www.feeddemon.com/ and http://net-newswireapp.com/ from Newsgator).

In order to make your feeds customized, you can add them to folders or categories you create such as "Medical News", "Medical Blogs" or "Favorite Websites". After clicking on "Organize" in the left sidebar, these folders can be created by choosing the "New Category" button.

Creating RSS Feed for Your Own Digital Channels

Most social media channels such as blog platforms or micro-blogging sites make the RSS feed of your channel available automatically, but in other cases custom RSS feed has to be created. Such services that convert your webpage or digital channel into a formatted RSS feed include Feed43 (http://www.feed43.com/) and Feedity (http://feedity.com/). After inserting the webpage URL of the desired dynamic content (e.g. new website, blog, audio/video content, or photostream, among others), the new RSS feed becomes available which you can publicize on your online channels.

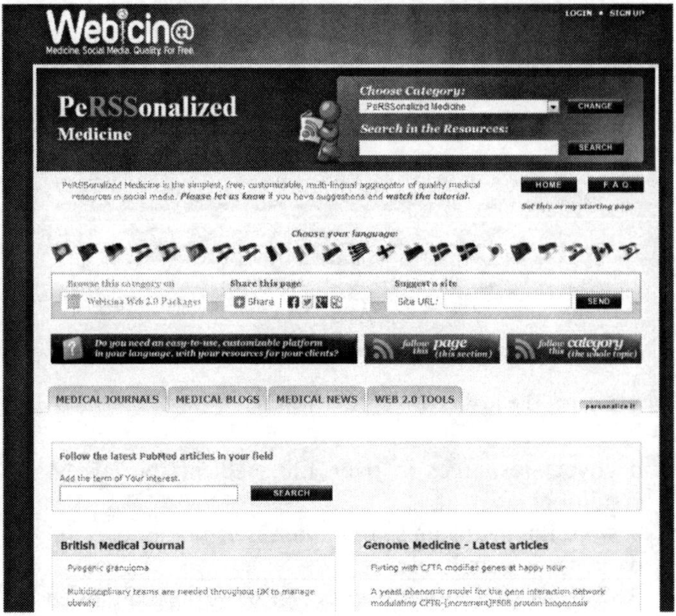

FIGURE 3.9 The main page of PeRSSonalized Medicine

Tracking Medical News, Websites and Social Media Resources

News tracker services aggregate the latest news items of different sources of information similarly to RSS readers but instead of users adding RSS feeds, these services contain pre-select news resources.

PeRSSonalized Medicine (http://www.webicina.com/perssonalized) curates medical peer reviewed and social media resources in a free aggregator with the following features (Fig. 3.9):

- customizable resource collection
- no registration needed
- multi-lingual meaning that national versions include resources from that language

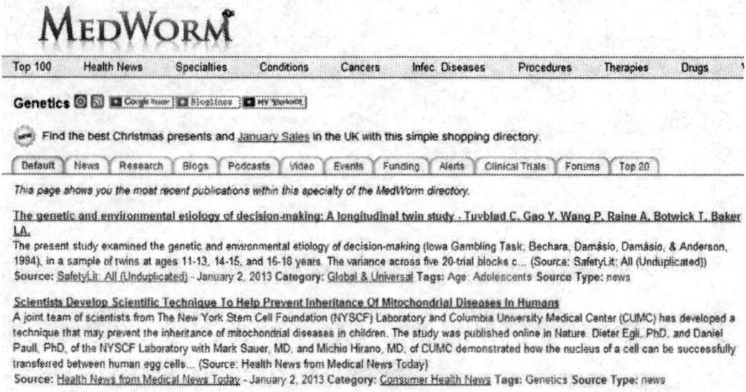

FIGURE 3.10 The main page of MedWorm

- it covers resources in over 130 medical specialties and conditions
- custom Pubmed.com search queries can be imported
- database is searchable
- RSS feeds of different topics can be exported and added to RSS readers

Medworm.com (http://www.medworm.com) serves as a router for medical RSS feeds as it aggregates all kind of RSS feeds into different categories but it does not allow customization and mostly excludes social media-related resources (Fig. 3.10).

Docphin (https://www.docphin.com/) focuses on medical research and full-text articles from peer reviewed papers but it requires institutional subscription.

The quality of news aggregators can be assessed based on:

- whether the source of the resources and the method by which they are selected are clearly defined
- information about the curators and authors of the aggregator is described
- contact information is available on the website
- dates are assigned to news items

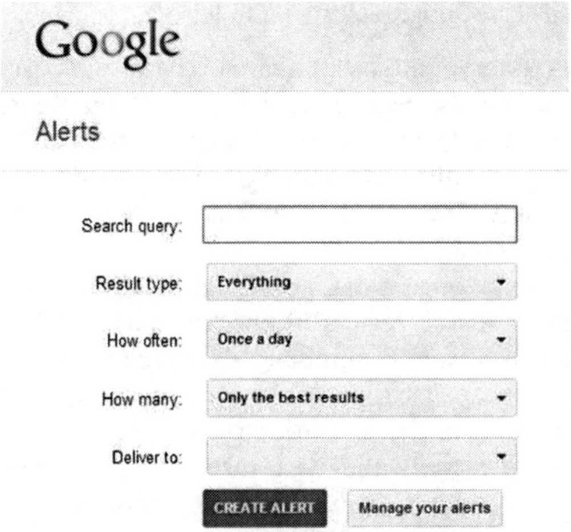

FIGURE 3.11 The dashboard of Google Alerts where details about e-mail alerts can be set (Google and the Google logo are registered trademarks of Google Inc., used with permission)

Creating Automated Search Alerts

Search alert tools send e-mail updates of the latest search results based on specific queries. Google Alerts (http://www.google.com/alerts) is a commonly used alert service for following news, websites and any kind of dynamic content appearing in the search engine of Google (Fig. 3.11). It is worth setting up automatic alerts for numerous queries:

- my name to see what websites mention it
- the name of my practice or clinic/institution
- fields of interest to keep myself up-to-date
- grant opportunities
- clinical guidelines

Settings for Google Alerts include:

- Search query: the basic search operators described in Chap. 2 can be used here such as "John Smith, MD", "link:www.website.com" or "diabetes AND cardiology".
- Result type: only news, only blogs, only videos, only discussions, only books or everything. The latter one is recommended.
- How often: "once a day" is recommended for terms that appear in search results often, "once a week" is recommended if a weekly summary of search results are sufficient; and "as-it-happens" is a recommended choice in case of important information such as our name.
- How many: "only the best results" is a recommended option for search queries probably resulting in a lot of results, while "all results" can be chosen if the expected amount of search results is manageable.
- Deliver to: it described which e-mail address the results will be delivered to.

After setting these details, the "Create alert" button will set it up, and the "Manage alerts" page will let you change the settings of different alerts or delete them. Fine-tuning the settings of the alerts is recommended after receiving the first few editions.

Receiving Automatic Alerts of New Citations of Biomedical and Scientific Papers

A "My citations" button in the right sidebar of Google Scholar allows the creation of a researcher profile. Research profiles have a "Follow new citations" option which sets up an automatic e-mail alert about new citations referring to the researcher (Fig. 3.12).

Self-Test

1. What kind of resources can be aggregated and syndicated through RSS?

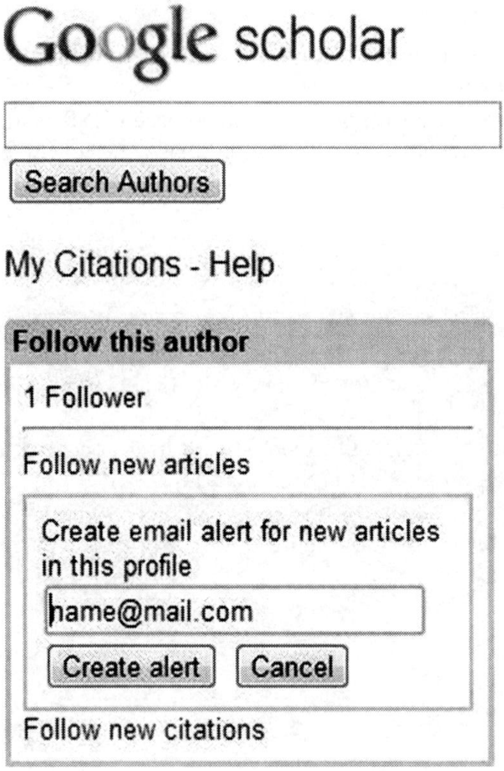

Google scholar

Search Authors

My Citations - Help

Follow this author

1 Follower

Follow new articles

Create email alert for new articles
in this profile

hame@mail.com

Create alert   Cancel

Follow new citations

FIGURE 3.12 E-mail alerts on Google Scholar (Google and the Google logo are registered trademarks of Google Inc., used with permission)

Any dynamic resources such as news, photos, blogs, podcast, video channels, etc.

2. How can I subscribe to the RSS feed of a resources such as a blog?

By inserting the RSS feed which can be accessed by clicking on the RSS feed icon into the RSS reader.

3. For what search queries should I set up e-mail alerts?

Our name, the name of our practice or clinic/institution, fields of interest; grant opportunities and clinical guidelines, among others.

Next Steps

- Try to find the RSS icons and feeds of your favorite online resources.
- Choose a web, mobile or desktop based RSS reader.
- Add a few RSS feeds to the database and let the information come to you.

Key Points

- RSS is a tool for delivering news and updates of dynamic resources to one RSS reader.
- RSS feeds can be read in web-, desktop- and mobile based RSS readers.
- Subscribing to the feeds of medical news and peer-reviewed papers is simple and free.
- E-mail alerts can be set up to receive updates about websites mentioning our name, workplace or field of interest.

References

1. Johnson SM, et al. Developing a current awareness service using really simple syndication (RSS). J Med Libr Assoc. 2009;97(1):52–4.
2. Ovadia S, et al. Staying informed with really simple syndication (RSS). Behav Soc Sci Libr. 2012;31(3–4):179–83.

Chapter 4
Community Sites: Facebook, Google+ and Medical Social Networks

Practicing medicine is teamwork. While 86 % of medical professionals use the Internet to access health information, 92 % of them access it from their office [1]; and 71 % of them use community sites [2]. One of the main reasons for using a community sites is that the person with the right answer for our question is not always present in the clinical setting therefore turning to the online world is a fast and potentially accurate alternative, although it has limitations.

Community sites usually bear with the following features:

- users have to register through a login system
- users can create profiles for themselves
- users can submit content including text or media files
- users can comment on each other's content
- groups can be created
- private and public messaging is possible
- users can search in the submitted content

There are potential advantages and disadvantages of using community sites for professional purposes (Table 4.1).

Basically there are two types of community sites which medical professionals can use for work-related purposes such as medical and non-medical community sites. Differences between the two types are summarized in Table 4.2.

B. Meskó, *Social Media in Clinical Practice*,
DOI 10.1007/978-1-4471-4306-2_4,
© Springer-Verlag London 2013

TABLE 4.1 Potential advantages and disadvantages of using community sites in medicine

Potential advantages	Potential disadvantages
Accessing information quickly	Accuracy of information is questionable
Finding new contacts	Each user profile has to be assessed
Free to use	Users are hardly motivated to contribute
Information is stored	Storage must comply with laws
Clinical cases can be shared	Privacy rights of patients might be compromised

TABLE 4.2 Differences between medical and non-medical community sites

	Community sites	Medical community sites
Registration	Anyone can register	Only medical professionals and students can register who must provide credentials
Focus areas	Non-specific	It can be medical specialty-specific
Language	Usually English	It can be language or country-specific
Policy	Common privacy policy	Privacy policy with a special focus on the Health Insurance Portability and Accountability Act

Non-medical Community Sites

Using Facebook as a Medical Professional

Facebook (http://www.facebook.com) is the world's largest community site with over one billion users [3]. Users have to register and create a personal profile, after which they can connect or "become friends" with other users, exchange messages and become members of groups or followers of pages. Based on a survey of 4,000 physicians, 61 % of them use Facebook for personal; and 15 % of them use it for professional purposes. Moreover, 33 % of physicians have received friend requests from their patients on Facebook and only 75 % of them declined the request [4]. Therefore the basic technical details and privacy issues have to be discussed.

Status updates as text messages, links, photos and videos can be shared on the timeline of a user which are meant to be seen only by the friends of the user which is not always the case. Even if the professional and personal lives are separated on Facebook, users should be aware of all the privacy settings that can be accessed under Settings – Privacy settings.

Details users should check before using Facebook:

- Who can see the content the user publishes (anyone, only friends, only the user or only customized groups).
- Whether the content the user was tagged in is published on the user's timeline without review.
- Who can look the user up using the e-mail address and phone number provided in the profile.
- Whether the timeline of the users appears in search engines.
- Who can publish content on the user's timeline.

If Facebook is used for professional purposes, the following settings are recommended to be used.

- Secure browsing should be used which can be accessed via Settings – Security.
- Only friends should see the content the user publishes.
- Content in which the user is tagged in should be reviewed before appearing on the timeline.
- Only friends should be able to look the user up using the e-mail address and phone number provided in the profile.
- The profile should not appear in search engines.
- Nobody should be allowed to publish content on the user's timeline.

Before a user posts content on the timeline, the people the content is shared with can be set through a small icon below the post (Table 4.3).

Facebook applications usually require access to the timeline, messages, friend list or even more details of the user,

TABLE 4.3 Privacy settings of posts published on Facebook

The setting of the post	The content is shared with
Public	Anyone
Friends	Only those users we became friends with
Only me	Only the user who made the post
Custom	A specified group of users
Groups	Existing groups
Friends of friends	The group of users cannot be specified

therefore the list of apps that have been given such access should be reviewed and access should be revoked via Settings – Apps settings.

In order to make sure only a specified group of users can see the post published by us, groups can be created under Groups – Create a group. The group must be named and members can be added immediately out of the friends the user already has. There are three options for the privacy settings of the group such as open (anyone can see the group, its members and the posts); closed (anyone can see the group and its members, but only members can see the posts); and secret (only members can see the group, its members and the posts).

For medical groups, the secret option should be chosen.

> **What if a Patient Sends a Friendship Request to His/Her Doctor on Facebook?**
> If the doctor's Facebook profile is personal, the request should be declined and a private message should be sent to the patient explaining the reasons. As the patient-doctor relationship is professional, it should not be mixed with a personal online profile.

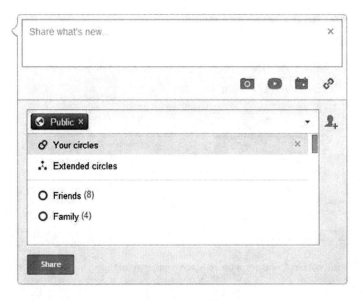

FIGURE 4.1 Privacy settings of posts on Google+

Using Google+ for Medical Purposes

Google+ (http://plus.google.com) is the community site launched by Google in 2011 having over 500 million registered users. It is described by Google as a social layer consisting of several layers that cover the online services and properties of Google. A clear difference compared to Facebook is the way Google+ makes it simple to use privacy settings while publishing content on the site.

Groups of users are called circles and can be created and defined by users. Posts can be shared with anyone (public), specific users or specific circles (Fig. 4.1).

Communities are the equivalent of Facebook groups in which users can follow ongoing conversations about particular topics. Communities can be public and private which only allows invited members to join the community and see the content. If public is chosen, it has to be decided

What kind of community are you making?

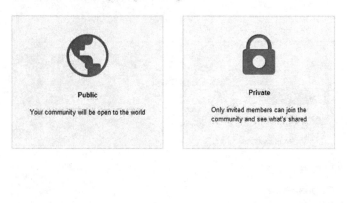

FIGURE 4.2 Creating a Google+ community

whether users need permission to join the community. If the private option is chosen, it has to be defined whether users can search for the community and ask for permission to join (Fig. 4.2).

Google Hangouts facilitate group video chat and can be launched by Google+ users. There are regular international clinical case presentations initiated via Google Hangouts which can easily be used for such purposes.

Using LinkedIn for Maintaining Professional Relationships

LinkedIn (http://www.linkedin.com) is a social networking site launched in 2003 intended for people in professional occupations and contact with any user requires an existing relationship which is meant to build trust among users.

Curriculum vitaes can be uploaded including workplaces, profile image, education, experience, awards, skills, interests and recommendations. A public profile with a short link can be created when the curriculum vitae is successfully uploaded. This link can substitute an own website as well.

Using Groups on Friendfeed for Archived Communication

FriendFeed (http://www.friendfeed.com) is a real-time aggregator of updates from social media resources such as blogs, community sites or microblogging services, among others. Groups related to specific topics can be created such as the Doctors, Students, & Health Care Professionals group launched for the blogs, Twitter feeds and other channels of medical professionals and students.

Medical Community Sites

There are community sites specifically created by and for medical professionals. These sites require credentials or copy of diploma during registration and content published on the social networks can only be accessed by registered users (Table 4.4).

Choosing the right community site is not an easy decision but numerous factors can facilitate this process such as:

- language of the social networking site
- the main topics it covers (research or medical specialties)
- the size of the community
- whether images, videos and clinical cases can be uploaded
- the privacy settings (how closed the community is)

The key factors when using medical or non-medical community sites are that patient privacy when clinical cases are shared should be respected and privacy settings should be analyzed in details.

A typical registration process is shown by using the example of Sermo, a US based community site. Users must specify their credential, name, e-mail address, street address, city, state, zip code, date of birth and the last four digits of the social security number.

TABLE 4.4 Medical community sites

Name and URL of social network	Basic features	Topics or specialty
Ozmosis (http://www.ozmosis.com)	A private and secure community for US based physicians	Not specialty-based
Dxy (http://www.dxy.cn)	A Chinese community with over two million members	Not specialty-based
Sermo (http://www.sermo.com)	The largest US based community	Not specialty-based
Doctors Hangout (http://www.doctorshangout.com)	A professional community with personal activities involved	Not specialty-based
Doctors.net.uk (http://www.doctors.net.uk)	The largest UK based medical community site	Not specialty-based
Nature Network (http://network.nature.com)	A social networking site for scientists organized by Nature.com	Not specialty-based
CMA (http://www.cma.ca)	Canadian medical community	Not specialty-based
EchoJournal (http://www.echjournal.org)	Video channel and community about echocardiology	Echocardiography
New Media Medicine (http://www.newmediamedicine.com)	A New Zealand based community site	Not specialty-based
Doctrs (http://www.doctrs.com)	A community site for finding coworkers and colleagues	Not specialty-based
Medcrowd (http://www.medcrowd.com)	A medical community for everyone working in healthcare	Not specialty-based
Esanum (http://www.esanum.com)	A multi-lingual (German, French and Spanish) medical community	Not specialty-based

A few tips for assessing the quality of basically any types of online medical resources:

- It should be easy to find out who runs the website
- It should be clear who pays for the website or if it is non-profit
- The purpose/mission statement of the website should be described
- The original source of the website's information should be available
- It should be easy to tell where the information comes from
- Time and date of the articles as well as the information included in them should be stated

Self-Test

1. Is using community sites as doctors safe?
   If the professional and personal profiles are separated and it is used with strategy, it should be safe.
2. What are the main differences between medical and non-medical community sites?
   Medical ones require credentials at registration and has features specifically designed for medical professionals.
3. What are the most popular community sites?
   Facebook, Google+, and LinkedIn.

Next Steps

1. Check your already existing profiles in social networking sites and see whether you mix personal and professional content.
2. Check the list of medical community sites and see whether there are any of them being relevant to your needs, language or specialty.
3. Try to find medical groups on Facebook, Google+ and other non-medical social networks.

Key Points
- There are medical and non-medical community sites.
- Medical communities require credentials and only medical professionals can use them.
- Patients usually contact their physicians on non-medical communities such as Facebook or Google+.
- Professional and personal community profiles of medical professionals should be clearly separated.
- LinkedIn is a decent community site to publish an online CV.

References

1. Dolan, Pamela Lewis. 2010. 86 % of physicians use Internet to access health information. http://www.ama-assn.org/amednews/2010/01/04/bisc0104.htm. Accessed 28 Jan 2013.
2. Taking the Pulse® U.S. http://manhattanresearch.com/Products-and-Services/Physician/Taking-the-Pulse-U-S. Accessed 28 Jan 2013.
3. Facebook: One Billion and Counting. http://online.wsj.com/article/SB10000872396390443635404578036164027386112.html. Accessed 28 Jan 2013.
4. Facebook has 845 million monthly users, and other interesting S-1 facts. http://thenextweb.com/facebook/2012/02/01/facebook-has-845-million-monthly-users-and-other-interesting-s-1-facts/. Accessed 28 Jan 2013.

Chapter 5
The World of E-Patients

Patients are motivated to get the information they need about their diagnoses or treatments, and turning to the Internet for accessing such information is inevitable. The number of e-patients is rapidly growing [1], and medical professionals must be able to respond to their special questions about health and the Internet which means specific skills have to be acquired.

The features of a good patient of the future were described in 2003 as follows [2]:

- Prepare a list of questions before the consultation.
- Want to share medical decisions with their healthcare providers.
- Need access to their electronic health records.
- Request a second opinion when facing a major decision.
- Use digital technologies for accessing health information.

Such good patients can be powerful agents initiating a change in the way healthcare is delivered and medicine is practiced. Medical professionals need to know how patients use online and mobile technologies; and how they use it in their decision making in order to make them equal partners in the care.

Basically, patients have been divided into three groups such as the "internal controller" who believes they are in charge of their own future health; the "external controller" who does not believe they have any control over their health;

B. Meskó, *Social Media in Clinical Practice*,
DOI 10.1007/978-1-4471-4306-2_5,
© Springer-Verlag London 2013

TABLE 5.1 The differences between Googlers and E-patients

Features	Googlers	E-patients
Use digital technologies in their health management	Yes	Yes
Use the Internet with strategy	No	Yes
Can deal with the huge amount of online information	No	Yes
Relationship with their doctor	Frustrating	Equal partners

and the "powerful other" who believes the doctor alone is in charge of their health [3]. Based on the e-patient movement, patients start preferring the "internal controller" type and want to be involved in decisions about their health but via different ways.

Patients who use the Internet without strategy or the required skills and take all the search results they find to their doctors are sometimes referred to as Googler patients or cyberchondriacs [4], while those patients using the Internet with strategy and asking the opinion of their medical professionals about the content they find online can be equal partners. Obviously there are a pieces of information available online but it is an expert's responsibility and duty to find out what to ignore. The main differences and similarities between Googlers and e-patients are summarized in Table 5.1.

E-patients or Internet patients are health consumers using the Internet and digital technologies for gathering information about a medical condition or treatment [5]. Research has shown that e-patients have "better health information and services, and different (but not always better) relationships with their doctors" [6].

Basic features of e-patients include the following factors.

- equipped with the skills to manage their own condition
- enabled to make choices about self-care
- empowered to make decisions together with their medical professionals
- engaged in their own care

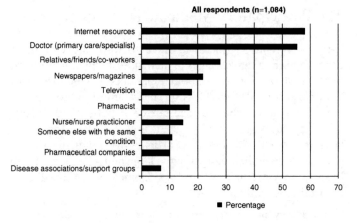

All respondents (n=1,084)

Internet resources
Doctor (primary care/specialist)
Relatives/friends/co-workers
Newspapers/magazines
Television
Pharmacist
Nurse/nurse practicioner
Someone else with the same condition
Pharmaceutical companies
Disease associations/support groups

0 10 20 30 40 50 60 70

■ Percentage

FIGURE 5.1 Resources of information patients find reliable (*Source*: [7])

- equals in their partnerships with the medical professionals involved in their care
- emancipated
- experts of their own condition

A few numbers and statistics describe the changes healthcare has to deal with due to the rising number of e-patients [1] (Fig. 5.1):

- 80 % of Internet users (61 % of all adults) search online to find health information
- 60 % of them consume social media and 29 % contributed content
- 19 % consult physician reviews, 18 % consult reviews of hospitals
- 60 % of e-patients say the information found online affected a decision about how to treat a medical condition
- 56 % say it changed their overall approach to their health management
- 53 % say it lead them to ask a doctor new questions or get second opinion
- 38 % say it affected a decision whether to see a doctor

The Participatory Medicine Movement

E-patients realized that they have to form movements in order to initiate real changes in medicine and healthcare. One of the first white papers about e-patients was published by Tom Ferguson, MD in 2007 [8]. The group of authors focusing on this topic grouped together on E-patients.net (http://www.e-patients.net) and launched a group blog. The group later found The Society for Participatory Medicine (http://participatorymedicine.org/) and launched the Journal of Participatory Medicine (http://www.jopm.org/). According to their mission statement [9]:

> The Society for Participatory Medicine is a 501(c)3 public charity devoted to promoting the concept of *participatory medicine* by and among patients, caregivers and their medical teams and to promote clinical transparency among patients and their physicians through the exchange of information, via conferences, as well through the distribution of correspondence and other written materials.

Resources and Platforms E-Patients Use

E-patients are web-savvy and try to find those resource, platforms and online channels that serve them best. Resources e-patients can use are summarized in an exemplary topic such as fitness (Table 5.2).

Besides blogs, Youtube channels or Twitter channels, forums and community sites attract and motivate most patients. Patientslikeme (http://www.patientslikeme.com/) is one of the first examples for a community sites used by patients. It was found in 2005 with a focus on Amyotrophic lateral sclerosis, but later became open to any conditions. It provided the platform for the first online clinical trial of which the results were published in a peer reviewed journal [10]. It now has several collaboration partnerships with research and academic institutions. In 2011, it announced the release of a tool which show a list of trials from ClinicalTrials.gov

TABLE 5.2 Type of social media resources e-patients use in a particular topic

Name of the resource	Type of the resource
Get Fit Slowly (http://getfitslowly.com/)	Blog
Dr Fitness and The Fat Guy (http://www.drfitnessandthefatguy.com)	Podcast
Fitness Wiki (http://fitness.wikia.com)	Wiki
Fitness Town (https://twitter.com/FitnessTown)	Twitter channel
Fitness on Slideshare.net	Slideshows
Fitness Builder (https://www.fitnessbuilder.com)	Mobile application
Vanity Health Club (http://www.youtube.com/user/VanityHealthClubs)	Youtube channel

TABLE 5.3 Medical community sites designed for patients

Name of the community site	Medical conditions it is related to
Patientslikeme (http://www.patientslikeme.com/)	Any conditions
Inspire (http://www.inspire.com)	Any conditions
MD Junction (http://www.mdjunction.com)	Any conditions
Autism One (http://www.autismone.org)	Autism
Cancer Forward (http://www.cancerforward.org/)	Cancer
D Life (http://www.dlife.com/)	Diabetes
Baby Center (http://www.babycenter.com)	Pregnancy
Crohnology (http://crohnology.com/)	Crohn's disease

to their members specific to their medical condition and demographics [11].

Examples are shown in Table 5.3.

E-Patient Stories

Story #1: Maarten Lens-FitzGerald is a Dutch patient who discovered he had a tumor between his lungs and decided to write a blog (http://maartensjourney.wordpress.com/) from the diagnosis through the treatment in order to get feedback from around the world. He was advised in a comment of his blog to contact a US-based oncologist and he connected his oncologist with him. The US oncologist made suggestions about the treatment, and Maarten published a blog entry stating that he was cancer free in 2009. He reported his blog helping a lot in his recovery.

Story #2: Erin Turner had immense pain in her right hand for a long time when she heard about an upcoming open discussion with Mayo clinic hand specialist, Dr. Richard Berger, on Twitter which she joined and got in touch with Dr. Berger. She was advised to travel to Mayo Clinic and had a surgery to correct the problem which turned out to be a solution for her medical issue [12].

Story #3: Kerri Morrone Sparling launched a blog in 2005 (http://sixuntilme.com/) about her own battle with diabetes. Throughout the years, she became a key voice in the medical blogosphere and leader of huge online diabetes communities. She inspires not only fellow patients, but medical professionals as well.

Story #4: Lauren Parrott was diagnosed with Multiple Sclerosis at the age of 18 and launched a Youtube video channel (http://www.youtube.com/user/laurenvparrott) in her twenties in order to share her insights and experience with the disease with the public and fellow patients. Her Youtube channel has over 1,800 subscribers and over half a million video views.

Story #5: "e-Patient Dave" deBronkart was diagnosed with Stage IV renal cell carcinoma in January 2007 and by September it was clear he had beaten the disease also due to the information he found online. He started writing a blog (http://epatientdave.com/) and was one of the first initiators of the e-patient movement. He is now a world-famous patient advocate and leader of the e-patient movement.

Story #6: Corey and Ellen Menscher designed and developed a device that alerts Twitter each time the baby kicked when Ellen was pregnant (http://kickbee.net). The patent of the baby kick detector is currently pending.

Dealing with Googlers and E-Patients

As patients do not learn how to use the web efficiently, it is possible that in most cases doctors will first face Googlers who find a lot of information online and become frustrated as they do not know how to deal with that making their own doctors frustrated too. The task of the medical professionals of the 21st century is to transform Googlers into e-patients with a few targeted questions.

Here is a potential scenario:

- Patient: "I found websites about my condition by using Google".
- Doctor: "On what website did you find the information?"
- Patient: "Here is the address of the website."
- Doctor: "Did you see the HONcode, Webicina or Healthcare Blogger Code of Ethics logo on the website?"
- Patient: "No."
- Doctor: "Then you cannot be sure that website is medically reliable, but here are two great resources written by professionals and fellow patients about your condition that I recommend reading."

E-Patient Dave deBronkart provided practical pieces of advice about dealing with e-patients in his book [13] (Fig. 5.2):

> My view: patients are the ultimate stakeholders – the ones who live or die, suffer or improve, based on how it all works out. In my view, treatment goals should arise in discussion between clinicians and patients. And if *I'm* the one who sets the goal of the treatment, I call it **achievement**, not behaving myself!

It is possible to describe the information for the patients without jargons; using reliable online resources and clear explanations. This is the responsibility of doctors to know at least two to three online resources in every condition they

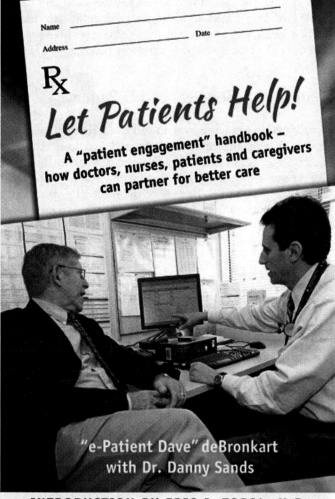

FIGURE 5.2 The cover of Let Patients Help author by E-Patient Dave deBronkart

deal with. Medical professionals should act as sentries of online information, as well as helpful producers/enablers of online resources.

Self-Test

1. Who are e-patients?
   E-patients use the information found online in their health management with strategy.
2. Why should Googlers be transformed into e-patients?
   Because e-patients can be equal partners in the treatment with good communication.
3. What is the name of the movement initiated by e-patients?
   Participatory medicine.

Next Steps

1. Ask your patients whether they look for and if so, how they find information online.
2. Know the digital space focusing on your field of interest and/ or specialty and know a few top quality resources by heart.
3. Check out Webicina, HONcode and other quality assessment tools therefore you can advise your patients which resource to choose.

Key Points
- Patients are motivated to use the Internet in their own health management.
- But being an e-patient means using digital technologies with strategy.
- E-patients use a whole spectrum of social media resources and channels.
- Googler patients should be transformed into e-patients with a few targeted questions.

References

1. The Rise of the e-Patient. http://www.pewinternet.org/Presentations/2012/Jan/The-Rise-of-the-ePatient.aspx. Accessed 28 Jan 2013.
2. Jadad AR, et al. I am a good patient, believe it or not. BMJ. 2003;326(7402):1293–5. http://www.ncbi.nlm.nih.gov/pmc/articles/PMC1126181/.

3. Different Types of Patients. http://ezinearticles.com/?Different-Types-of-Patients&id=411496. Accessed 28 Jan 2013.
4. Cyberchondria.   http://en.wikipedia.org/wiki/Cyberchondria. Accessed 28 Jan 2013.
5. E-patient. http://en.wikipedia.org/wiki/E-patient. Accessed 20 Jun 2013.
6. Internet Health Resources. http://www.pewinternet.org/~/media// Files/Reports/2003/PIP_Health_Report_July_2003.pdf.pdf. Accessed 28 Jan 2013.
7. How America Searches. http://www.icrossing.com/sites/default/files/ how-america-searches-health-and-wellness.pdf. Accessed 28 Jan 2013.
8. E-patients white paper. http://e-patients.net/e-Patients_White_ Paper.pdf. Accessed 28 Jan 2013.
9. Society for Participatory Medicine. http://participatorymedicine.org/ about/. Accessed 28 Jan 2013.
10. Wicks P, et al. Accelerated clinical discovery using self-reported patient data collected online and a patient-matching algorithm. Nat Biotechnol. 2011;29:411–4.
11. Patientslikeme Launches New Feature For Patients To Accelerate Clinical Trials Enrollment. http://www.patientslikeme.com/ press/20110609/28-patientslikeme-launches-new-feature-for-patients-to-accelerate-clinical-trial-enrollment. Accessed 28 Jan 2013.
12. My E-Patient Twitter Success Story. http://www.spectrumscience. com/blog/2010/02/26/my-e-patient-twitter-success-story/. Accessed 28 Jan 2013.
13. Let Patients Help!. https://www.createspace.com/3682541. Accessed 26 Mar 2013.

Chapter 6
Establishing a Medical Blog

Social media brought a new concept into the online world as users became able to contribute content to websites. One of the first platforms that made this possible was called a blog. A blog is a website with regular entries of commentary or other materials such as graphics or video displayed in a reverse chronological order. The term blog was first used by Jorn Barger in 1997 from the words we – blog or web – log [1] (Fig. 6.1).

Definitions of expressions related to a blog:

- Blog post or entry: The item published with text and/or media materials.
- Comment: A message left on a specific entry.
- Tag: A category used for the entry to make it easy to find it later.
- Blogroll: A list of blogs the author of the blog likes or endorses.
- Trackback: A method for website authors to request notification when another blog links to one of the entries.

A medical professionals can express opinions or commentaries on their blogs they could never do in official or scientific channels. There are different types of blogs (Table 6.1).

The quality of a blog can be assessed by numerous features such as whether contact details, author information, blog description, archive, privacy policy and medical disclaimer are available. But the popularity of the blog, the number of entries published or the credentials of authors do not determine the blog's quality.

B. Meskó, *Social Media in Clinical Practice*,
DOI 10.1007/978-1-4471-4306-2_6,
© Springer-Verlag London 2013

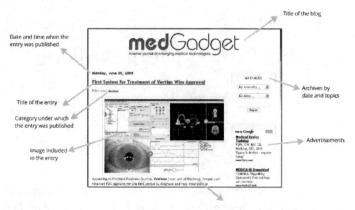

FIGURE 6.1 The anatomy of a medical blog

TABLE 6.1 The types of blogs

Type of blog	Its focus or special feature	An example
Photoblog	Photos	http://www.dianevarner.com/
Personal blog	Personal life	http://theinterpreterdiaries.com/
Group blog	The blog has several authors	http://www.medgadget.com
Company blog	The blog is the company's channel	http://www.blogsouthwest.com
Videoblog	Videos	http://coachtvblog.com/
Tematic blog	Specific topics	http://streetanatomy.com/

Researchers are advised to engage with the blogosphere [2]:
"More researchers should engage with the blogosphere, including authors of papers in press."

Since August of 2007, blogs can be cited in peer reviewed papers using the guidelines of The National Library of Medicine and National Institute of Health [3] (Fig. 6.2).

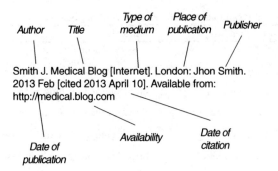

FIGURE 6.2 The way of citing medical blogs in medical papers

The Medical Blogosphere

All stakeholders of healthcare can write blogs and present their own areas, research topics or job experience from their own perspectives. The table summarizes the different types of medical blogs with examples (Table 6.2).

Kovic et al., analyzed the medical blog world (blogosphere) and identified key elements about how the medical blog network works and what the bloggers are like [4].

- 58 % of medical bloggers are 30–49 years old
- 59 % of them are male
- 35 % of them are doctors
- 56 % of them spend more than 20 h a week online
- 96 % use broadband connection
- 99, 86 and 66 % of them read medical news online, on blogs, and with RSS, respectively
- 24 % listen to medical news via podcasts
- 25 % of them blog anonymously
- 54 % of them have scientific publications

After a few years of blogging, blog carnivals were created in order to select the most important blog entries about a particular topic every week on one selected blog. The original and still ongoing blog carnival is called Grand Rounds and features medical blogs in any relevant topics [5]. Other blog

TABLE 6.2 Examples of different kinds of medical blogs

Type of medical blog	Example
Nurse blog	http://www.codeblog.com/
Doctor blog	http://www.familymedicinerocks.com/
Medical student blog	http://internal-optimist.blogspot.com
Medical lawyer blog	http://lawmedconsultant.com/
Hospital manager blog	http://runningahospital.blogspot.com
Medical librarian blog	http://laikaspoetnik.wordpress.com/
Patient blog	http://sixuntilme.com/

carnivals were also launched later such as Gene Genie in genetics or Medicine 2.0 in digital medical communication. The majority of blog carnivals were transformed into micro-blogs from 2011.

Reasons to Write a Blog

A blog can be a useful channel for making new contacts worldwide and for building an online reputation. Alan J. Cann uses his microbiology blog for keeping in touch with his medical students (http://scienceoftheinvisible.blogspot.com). Being active in the medical blogosphere may lead to discovering new ways for international collaboration, lead to better writing skills; and learn to reach people with a new form of communication.

Positive and negative stories represent the real value and potential legal limitations of medical blogging:

Story #1: Two American molecular and cell biology graduate students launched a blog under the name NCBI ROFL in which they started collecting scientific papers presenting special and strange research topics. Later the blog was transferred to the website of Discover (http://blogs.discovermagazine.com/discoblog).

Story #2: In 2008, Arnold Kim left practicing medicine to become a full time technology blogger on Macrumors.com [6].

Story #3: Dr Flea was a famous anonymous medical blogger in 2007–2008, but the author got sued in his practice and

TABLE 6.3 The 7 basic types of bloggers

Type of blogger	Features of the type
The Barber	Knows the right people and information.
The Blacksmith	Like the Barber but blogging in a company.
The Bridge	Making new connection between people and topics.
The Window	Blogs about a company as an employee.
The Signpost	Points out interesting things in their topic.
The Pub	Creates discussions among people.
The Newspaper	Reports on new things as a journalist.

he kept on blogging about the lawsuit. The attorney found it out and the blog was deleted, Dr. Flea lost the lawsuit due to sharing "prior inconsistent statements" about the lawsuit publicly. He left his job. A similar story happened to the author of the WhiteCoat's Call Room blog, although he kept the HIPAA in mind while writing about the case and it did not cause any legal consequences to him [7].

Story #4: A Russian medical student was arrested as he started spreading rumors of a non-existing H1N1 "plague" on his medical blog for unknown reasons [8].

Story #5: The blogger of the Fauquier ENT blog described the reasons why he had been blogging such as being up-to-date by writing entries; marketing his own practice; and building credibility before the first meeting with the patient [9].

Steps to Make Before Launching a New Medical Blog

Three questions should be answered before launching a medical blog. (1) What kind of blogger would you be, (2) which platform would you choose for blogging, (3) how would you blog.

Step #1: There are seven basic types of bloggers as summarized in Table 6.3.

Step #2: Several free-to-use platforms can be used for blogging including Wordpress.com (http://www.wordpress.com), Blogger (http://www.blogger.com), and Typepad (http://www.typepad.com/). In quality, these are very close to each other, therefore it only depends on personal details which one is to be chosen. Wordpress is used as an example for launching a new blog.

The "Get Started" button leads to the registration page on Wordpress (Fig. 6.3).

Only a few details such as e-mail address, username, password and a blog address are required for launching a blog. A good blog address represents the topic of the blog is about; easy to remember and is appropriate for medical audiences (Fig. 6.4).

After registration, the dashboard becomes active where details about the blog including statistics, number of blog entries, tags, categories, recent posts and comments, among other are available (Fig. 6.5).

Choosing "Posts" – "Add new" leads to the edit view where new posts can be written (Fig. 6.6).

In order to write a new blog entry, a title of the post has to be given, the content whether it is text, video or photo

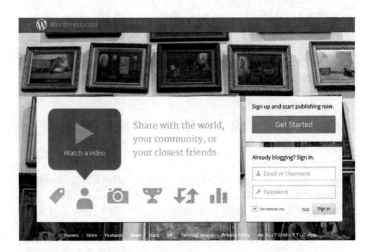

FIGURE 6.3   The main page of http://www.Wordpress.com

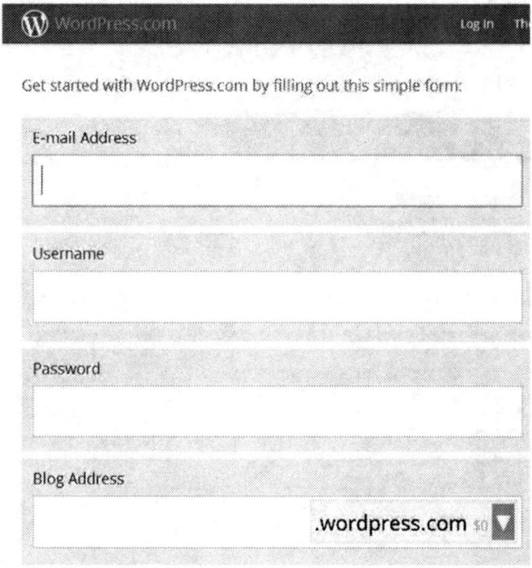

FIGURE 6.4 The four easy steps of creating a new blog on http://www.Wordpress.com

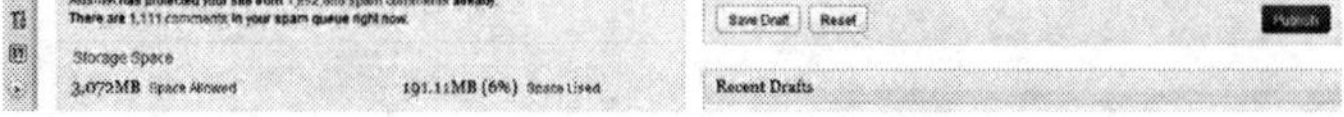

FIGURE 6.5 The dashboard of a blog hosted by http://www.Wordpress.com

can be inserted into the edit box, categories (for broader grouping of posts) and tags (similar to category but are generally used to describe the post in more details) can be added and the publish button makes it appear on the blog (Fig. 6.7). Posts can be scheduled in advance by using the Edit button next to Publish. If the post is saved as a draft, it can be accessed later from the dashboard and published.

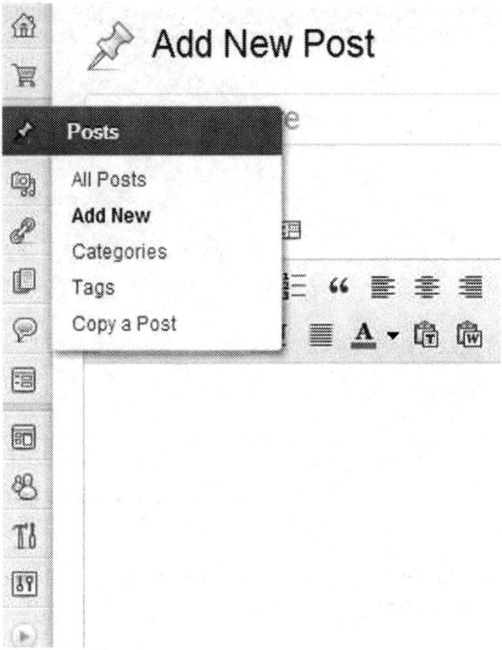

FIGURE 6.6 Creating a new blog entry on a blog hosted by http://www.Wordpress.com

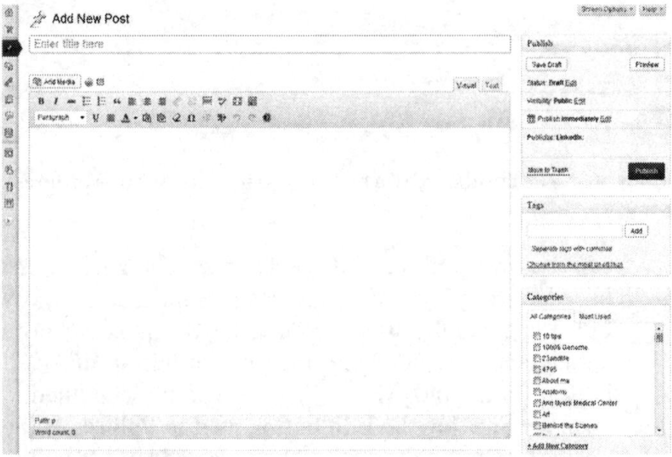

FIGURE 6.7 Creating a new blog entry on a blog hosted by http://www.Wordpress.com. The title, the text and the categories are shown

Features which are accessible from the left sidebar in the Dashboard:

- Posts: All the posts, categories and tags are available, and new post can be created.
- Media: The medical library and an option to add new media whether it is photo or video.
- Links: Links that appear in the blogroll can be checked and new ones added.
- Pages: All the pages with the option of adding a new page. Pages are static compared to blog entries which are dynamic.
- Comments
- Feedback: Polls and ratings can be created.
- Appearance: Themes, widgets, menus and background of the blog can be edited here.
- Users: New users can be added, roles can be defined and the admin's profile is accessible.
- Tools: The blog's content can be imported/exported or deleted.
- Settings: Details about reading, writing, discussing the blog, media, polls, advertisements, among others can be changed.

Step #3: Not only the content itself, but the way an author communicates will determine the success of the blog, therefore this is the key part in blogging. A few basic rules can assist in the process of becoming an experienced blogger:

- Openness: Being open to those who offer content/product reviews/interview opportunities to write about might lead to becoming the No. 1 target for these companies.
- Commitment: Be committed and work on your blog constantly, know your goals and evaluate often.
- Consistency: Choose a topic or some sub-topics to focus on and stick to your decision. In order to find the target audience, a blog needs a consistent topic.
- Before publishing an entry, the answer should be Yes for the following questions: is it OK if my patients/family members/friends/boss/employees see that?

Tips and Tricks About Making a Better Blog

There are several ways of improving the appearance or platform of your blog and make it easier for readers to assess its quality.

- An own logo gives a good picture about the blog if it represents the topic the blog discusses.
- Contact details should be added on the top of the sidebar (e-mail address as an image file in order to avoid our e-mail address getting into spam databases (http://services.nexodyne.com/email); Skype name, etc.)
- Odiogo creates automatic podcasts of your blog entries (http://www.odiogo.com/).
- Google Analytics (https://www.google.com/analytics) makes it easy to see where your readers are coming from and who they are.
- The license of the blog should be clearly described. Creative Commons provides a simple way of determining the license (http://creativecommons.org/). As blogs are about sharing, choosing a license that makes redistribution and share possible is recommended.

The Future of Blogging

While blogs will remain an important part of the user-generated content online, some blogs go through transitions. Personal diaries moved to Facebook, photoblogs moved to photo services such as Flickr.com, video blogs were transformed into Youtube channels and short discussions can now be found on microblogs such as Twitter.com.

Due to the amount of time and effort it takes to properly write a medical blog, some authors switch to writing microblogs on Tumblr.com.

Self-Test

1. What is a trackback?
   A method for website authors to request notification when another blog links to one of the entries.

2. How can the quality of a blog be assessed?
   With numerous features such as whether contact details, author information, blog description, archive, privacy policy and medical disclaimer are available.
3. What are the elements of the 3 rules of blogging?
   Openness, commitment and consistency.

Next Steps

1. Try to find blogs dedicated to your field of interest or specialty.
2. See whether there is a niche which you could fill in.
3. Choose a blog platform, make a well-established decision about the topics you would cover and type of blogger you would like to be and publish your first post.
4. Follow the 3 rules of medical blogging to get the best potential results.

Key Points
- A blog is a website with regular entries displayed in a reverse chronological order.
- Several healthcare professionals and patients write blogs.
- Choosing the platform and the type of communication, as well as following the 3 rules of blogging is important in writing quality blogs.

References

1. Jorn Barger. Weblog. http://en.wikipedia.org/wiki/Jorn_Barger#Weblog. Accessed 28 Jan 2013.
2. Editorial. It's good to blog. Nature. 2009;457:1058.
3. MLA Works Cited: Electronic Sources (Web Publications). http://owl.english.purdue.edu/owl/resource/747/08/. Accessed 28 Jan 2013.
4. Kovic I, et al. Examining the medical blogosphere: an online survey of medical bloggers. J Med Internet Res. 2008;10(3):e28.
5. Grand Rounds. http://getbetterhealth.com/grand-rounds. Accessed 28 Jan 2013.

6. My Son, the Blogger: An M.D. Trades Medicine for Apple Rumors. http://www.nytimes.com/2008/07/21/technology/21blogger.html?_r=1&oref=slogin. Accessed 28 Jan 2013.
7. Interview with Dr. Flea. http://scienceroll.com/2010/11/22/interview-with-dr-flea/. Accessed 28 Jan 2013.
8. Russia: Blogger Arrested For Pneumonic Plague Rumors. http://advocacy.globalvoicesonline.org/2009/12/04/russia-blogger-arrested-for-pneumonic-plague-rumors/. Accessed 28 Jan 2013.
9. As A Busy Physician, Why Do I Even Bother Blogging? http://fauquierent.blogspot.hu/2010/09/as-busy-physician-why-do-i-even-bother.html. Accessed 28 Jan 2013.

Chapter 7
The Role of Twitter and Microblogging in Medicine

As social media became widely popular through blogging and community sites, there was a clear need for a communication channel or platform that is fast, interactive and archived. The concept of using such a communication platform was not new as it was introduced in a train station in London, UK in 1935 [1] (Fig. 7.1). The user wrote a brief message on a continuous strip of paper and dropped a coin in the slot. The inscription moved up behind a glass panel where it remained in public view for at least 2 hours. The concept of microblogging is similar.

The most prominent example of microblogging is Twitter. com, a social networking service that enables users to send and read messages of up to 140 characters. It was launched in 2006 with a message posted by founder Jack Dorsey: "just setting up my twttr" [2]. The basic idea was to create the SMS of the Internet.

As of 2013, it has over 500 million users generating over 340 million messages per day [3]. Providing the user's full name, an e-mail address and password creates an account which is for free. Users receive the messages of other users they follow and vice versa (Fig. 7.2).

The settings make it possible to customize the account, and decide whether it should be protected (accessible only to those the user gives access to). The following elements can be accessed in settings:

- Account: basic, language and privacy settings.
- Password: password can be changed.
- Mobile: Mobile phone can be added to the account.

B. Meskó, *Social Media in Clinical Practice*,
DOI 10.1007/978-1-4471-4306-2_7,
© Springer-Verlag London 2013

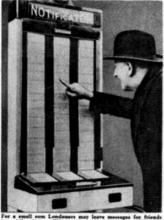

Robot Messenger Displays Person-to-Person Notes In Public

TO AID persons who wish to make or cancel appointments or inform friends of their whereabouts, a robot message carrier has been introduced in London, England.

Known as the "notificator," the new machine is installed in streets, stores, railroad stations or other public places where individuals may leave messages for friends.

The user walks up on a small platform in front of the machine, writes a brief message on a continuous strip of paper and drops a coin in the slot. The inscription moves up behind a glass panel where it remains in public view for at least two hours so that the person for whom it is intended may have sufficient time to observe the note at the appointed place. The machine is similar in appearance to a candy-vending device.

For a small sum Londoners may leave messages for friends in public places. When written on "notificator," message moves up behind window, remaining in view for two hours.

FIGURE 7.1 Robot messenger in a train station in London, UK, in 1935 (Used with permission from http://blog.modernmechanix.com/robot-messenger-displays-person-to-person-notes-in-public/)

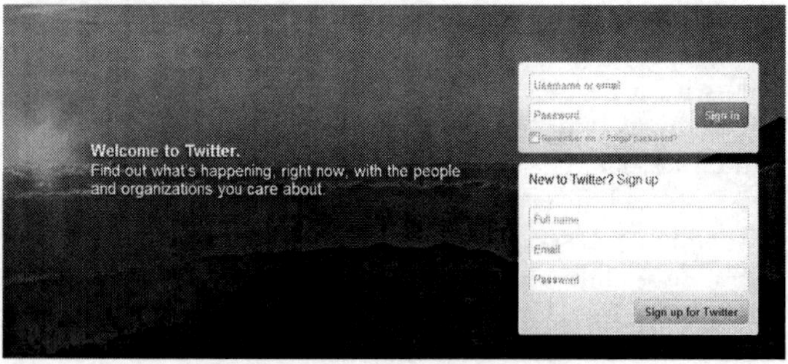

FIGURE 7.2 The main page of Twitter.com

- E-mail notification: It can be controlled when and how often Twitter sends e-mails.
- Profile: The most important element with the settings of the profile page.
- Design: Background image and profile picture can be uploaded.

- Apps: Applications being connected to the account.
- Widgets: Widgets can be added to the account.

Features that make a quality account:

- Full name should be given.
- A short biography with workplace.
- A website URL if available, or a LinkedIn profile.
- An appropriate profile image that accurately reflects your professional identity. It should look fine in thumbnail version as well.
- The Twitter account name should be easily recognizable containing only ten characters or less is recommended. Do not infringe on existing brands, avoid using nicknames or humorous names.

There are subpages of an account such as Home which shows the accounts the user follows; @Connect which shows the interactions with the user; #discover recommends users and tweets to follow; while Me directs to the profile of the user.

There are new definitions related to using Twitter:

- tweet: a message sent on Twitter containing no more than 140 characters.
- Twitterer: Twitter user.
- tweetchat or tweetup: a scheduled group discussion on Twitter.
- Followfriday: users recommend following other users by tagging them with #followfriday.
- hashtag: Expressions used to tag messages with topics such as #meded for medical education.

Communication on Twitter

Twitter is based on quick and interactive communication. To make sure the receiver receives a tweet, the user's name is inserted into the message following the @ sign.

"@Berci Here is my message."

This is also the way of replying to a user's tweet. Such tweets are publicly accessible. In order to send a private message which can only be seen by the recipient, direct messages can be used in which the user's name is placed after DM.

"DM Berci Here is my private message."

Messages can be tagged in order to manually label them with different topics or areas. Hashtags are inserted into messages for this purpose following the # sign.

"I wanted to share an article about high blood pressure treatment. #cardiology"

Accounts can be followed by clicking on the "Follow" button on the profile of the account; and unfollowed by clicking on the "unfollow" button.

Besides text, links, photos and videos as links can also be included in messages. Twitter has its own photo uploading service called Twitpic which is available when posting a message.

RT stands for retweet which means sharing someone else's tweet; while MT stands for modified tweet when the shared tweet is edited by the user.

Organizing Tweetchats

Twitter is suitable for structured discussions through conversations called tweetchats [4]. The following steps are required to create and organize a tweetchat:

1. A Twitter account has to be created with a name relevant to the topic or an existing account can be used.
2. A hashtag specific to the topic covered in the tweetchat should be designed.
3. Relevant content should be posted regularly in the account.
4. A regular day and time should be chosen for the tweetchats.
5. A website for archiving the text of the discussions is recommended.
6. Let participants send in questions before each meeting. Google Docs provides a good solution for that via a document that anyone can edit.

The First Steps After Creating an Account

1. Add a profile picture, biography, location and full name.
2. Search for topics of interest in the search box on Twitter. com.
3. It will list either relevant tweets or Twitterers.
4. Following them will provide relevant tweets.
5. Other target Twitter channels include news sources, professional associations and academic institutions of interest, clients, competitors and thought leaders.
6. The list of followers of the Twitter account which is of interest for us can lead to potentially interesting new Twitterers.
7. Twitscoop (http://www.twitscoop.com) refers to relevant topics, while Twellow (http://www.twellow.com) and WeFollow (http://www.wefollow.com) refer to potentially relevant Twitter users.
8. Providing quality content in a field of interest generally lead to new followers.
9. Using proper hashtags makes it easier to find relevant content (e.g. #hcsm for messages about healthcare and social media). Symplur (http://www.symplur.com/healthcare-hashtags/) collects healthcare-related hashtags.

Practical Details of Using Twitter

As tweets can only contain 140 characters, long website links (URLs) are advised to be shortened. The so-called URL shorteners such as http://www.bit.ly or http://www.ow.ly create short links.

Paper.li (http://www.paper.li) converts web content from Twitter or Facebook into an online newspaper. It uses hashtags or Twitter accounts as well.

Tweetdeck (http://www.tweetdeck.com) is a dashboard application that helps manage multiple Twitter accounts, replies/direct messages, search terms and hashtags (Fig. 7.3).

Tweets can be cited in medical papers as described by the Modern Language Association [5] (Fig. 7.4).

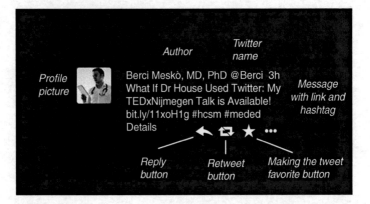

FIGURE 7.3 Tweetdeck aggregates all relevant tweets and makes it easy to reply easily

Last Name, First Name (User Name).
" The tweet in its entirety." Date, Time, Tweet.

FIGURE 7.4 The way of citing Twitter messages in academic publications

Potential Uses of Twitter in Medicine and Healthcare

While Twitter was not originally designed for medical purposes, there are numerous practical uses of it either for practices or hospitals, as well as in public health.

- Public health organizations send alerts about disasters and health issues.
- Drug safety alerts and announcements from FDA.
- Supportive care for patients.
- Live tweeting during medical conferences.
- Staying up-to-date.
- Hospitals using it for keeping in touch with patients.
- Hospitals tweeting live during operations [6].
- Crowdsourcing a diagnosis [7].
- Tracking the spread of disease in real time [8].
- Organizing medical tweetchats such as #medlib [9].
- Following users who can filter news in a specific field of interest.

TABLE 7.1 Examples of the different types of Twitter accounts

Type of Twitter account	Example
Organizations	https://twitter.com/WHOnews
Doctors	https://twitter.com/kevinmd
Medical journals	https://twitter.com/nejm
Hospitals	https://twitter.com/mayoclinic
Patients	https://twitter.com/sixuntilme

Figure: crisis communication by time

Several stakeholders of medicine and healthcare use Twitter for different purposes. Table 7.1 summarizes these examples.

Other Microblogging Platforms

Twitter is the most popular microblogging platform, though there are other solutions as well such as Friendfeed (http://www.friendfeed.com), or Tumblr (http://www.tumblr.com).

All these platforms feature medical pages, but most users focusing on medicine and healthcare are on Twitter.

Self-Test

1. What are the possible ways of communication on Twitter?
   Public and private messages.
2. What kind of content can be tweeted?
   Anything that can be represented as a URL.
3. What are the main microblogging platforms?
   Twitter, Friendfeed and Tumblr.

Next Steps

1. Do a search on Twitter for your field of interest and see whether there are users already covering this topic.
2. Start following them and if you would like to build an online profile for yourself by using Twitter, start sharing relevant content.
3. Be responsive, helpful and build your community wisely.

Key Points
- Twitter is a social networking service that enables users to send and read messages of up to 140 characters.
- It can be used for filtering news, being up-to-date or contacting colleagues worldwide.
- Organizations, medical journals and hospitals use Twitter for communication.
- Medical professionals should have an open account with clear description, affiliation and a real photo.

References

1. Robot Messenger Displays Person-to-Person Notes In Public (Aug, 1935). http://blog.modernmechanix.com/robot-messenger-displays-person-to-person-notes-in-public/. Accessed 28 Jan 2013.
2. Twitter's 5th birthday: five years since Jack Dorsey sent the first tweet. http://metro.co.uk/2011/03/21/twitters-5th-birthday-five-years-since-jack-dorsey-sent-the-first-tweet-645632/. Accessed 28 Jan 2013.
3. How to host a tweet chat on Twitter. http://stwem.com/2011/08/31/how-to-host-a-tweet-chat/. Accessed 28 Jan 2013.
4. Twitter on Wikipedia. http://en.wikipedia.org/wiki/Twitter. Accessed 28 Jan 2013.
5. How do I cite a tweet? http://www.mla.org/style/handbook_faq/cite_a_tweet. Accessed 28 Jan 2013.
6. Henry Ford Hospital Surgeons Twitter Surgery As Outreach & Teaching. http://etechlib.wordpress.com/2009/02/19/henry-ford-hospital-surgeons-twitter-surgery-as-outreach-teaching/. Accessed 28 Jan 2013.
7. From Twitter to the New York Times. http://scienceroll.com/2010/03/07/from-twitter-to-the-new-york-times/. Accessed 28 Jan 2013.
8. Twitter Revealed Epidemic Two Weeks Before Health Officials [STUDY]. http://mashable.com/2012/01/10/twitter-epidemic-choler-haiti/. Accessed 28 Jan 2013.
9. Medlibs Tweet Chat: Social Media. http://kraftylibrarian.com/?p=2121. Accessed 28 Jan 2013.

Chapter 8
Collaboration Online

It has never been that simple to collaborate without geographical limitations as the Internet brought us numerous tools and platforms that can facilitate this process. Before the Internet era, when manuscripts were written in large collaborations, the document was sent by post to the co-authors who made changes and sent the manuscript back to the main author, who created a new version which was sent out again. Mails back and forth in an inefficient, long, time-wasting process. E-mails made the process a bit faster, but co-authors still struggle to make it as efficient as possible [1, 2].

Saving time and effort is a key in the medical profession, therefore the use of convenient tools and platforms online for collaboration is recommended.

Things are advised to be considered before choosing an online resources for collaboration and these details should be described in advance.

- The number of users involved.
- Privacy of information, whether it should be public or private.
- Whether storage of data is needed.
- Whether recording of live talks is necessary.
- Whether the primary aim is discussion, live chat or project management.

B. Meskó, *Social Media in Clinical Practice*,   79
DOI 10.1007/978-1-4471-4306-2_8,
© Springer-Verlag London 2013

Group Discussions

The most popular software application for video chat is Skype (http://www.skype.com) with over 600 million registered members. After registration, it is possible to make international voice and video calls among users of Skype for free; as well as to make international phone calls and group video chat for a fee. While there were many case reports about using Skype in the healthcare settings, no evidence either in favour of, or against the use of it for clinical telehealth was found [3].

Other softwares which is free to use for non-commercial purposes are Mikogo (http://www.mikogo.com); or Oovoo (http://www.oovoo.com) which allows free video calls with up to 12 users. Google+ Hangouts are also used for group video chats (https://plus.google.com/u/0/hangouts).

FaceTalk (http://en.facetalk.nl/) was designed as a virtual consultation room for clinical purposes by the Radboud REshape & Innovation Center of the Netherlands. It was developed with clinical features in mind making group video chats or the transmission of medical file types possible and is available for a monthly fee (Fig. 8.1).

Written discussions are crucial in projects in which a written archive is important. Medical community sites primarily serve this purpose, while common social networks have features making such closed discussions possible such as closed groups on Facebook (http://www.facebook.com) which only invited users can join; medical groups of Friendfeed (http://www.friendfeed.com); Grouptweet which lets multiple users to contribute to one account (Fig. 8.2).

The opportunities of using online platforms for collaboration is endless including e-mail groups such as Googe Groups (http://groups.google.com); wikis for taking notes and collecting files shared by the group members such as Wikispaces (http://www.wikispaces.com/); but a blog or a Twitter account can also be used for this purpose.

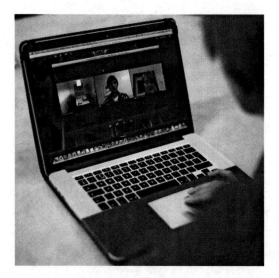

FIGURE 8.1 A screenshot about Facetalk

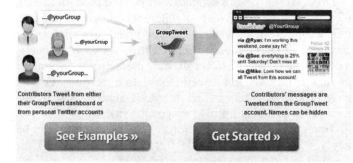

FIGURE 8.2 Grouptweet allows using the same Twitter account by different users

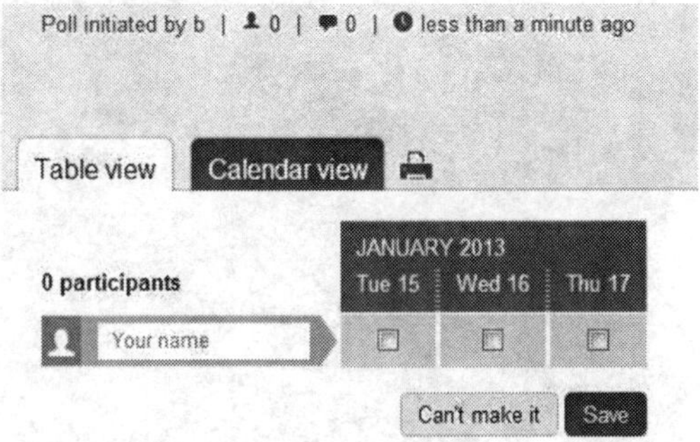

FIGURE 8.3 Doodle lets users add their names and choose dates and times suiting them best for a particular meeting

Tools for Project Management

Collaboration platforms are available for managing projects online such as creating tasks, appointments, notes and bookmarks, among others. Stixy (http://www.stixy.com) is an example for such purposes. Mindmeister (http://www.mindmeister.com) creates mind maps; and Cacoo (http://www.cacoo.com) creates online diagrams.

Dropbox (http://www.dropbox.com) can be used for sharing files or synchronizing folders of different computers. It offers a free account with a set storage size and paid subscriptions for accounts with more capacity. Scribd (http://www.scribd.com) is a document-sharing platform allowing users to post documents of various formats, and embed them into a webpage. Certain large files can also be sent and stored via common e-mail platforms such as Gmail (http://www.gmail.com).

Times and dates of discussions or online meetings can be easily scheduled with Doodle (http://www.doodle.com) for free through the following steps: (Fig. 8.3)

1. Choose the "Schedule an event" on the main page.
2. Provide a title, your name and e-mail address (description and location are optional).
3. Selecting dates and times within days.

4. It can be a basic poll, or a special one with more answer options or it can be hidden.
5. A URL of the poll is created which can be shared.

Writing Manuscripts Collaboratively

Google Docs (http://docs.google.com/) is a free web-based platform for working on documents, spreadsheets or presentations in a collaborative format as a part of the service of Google Drive (http://drive.google.com). It is a popular solution for working on a manuscript simultaneously [4]. The main features of Google Docs include:

- Each version of the document is automatically stored and can be accessed any time.
- Edits can be made in a simultaneous way.
- Specific edits are assigned to specific editors.
- The document can be published online or shared via e-mail.
- Colleagues can be added as editors who can edit the document, only comment on that or see that but cannot make edits.
- Documents can be exported in many file formats.
- Storage space is 5 GB (Google Docs formats do not count towards the storage limit).

Users can log into the dashboard of Google Docs by using a Google account and access the documents they have created or that have been shared with them. The title of the document, the owner's name, the date of the last modification; and whether the document was starred by the user are shown. Documents can be grouped by different parameters: all files; files shared with me; starred files; and files that were recently modified (Fig. 8.4).

New files or folders can be uploaded by using the upload sign next to the "Create" button. By clicking on the "Create" button, documents, presentations, spreadsheets, forms, drawings, folders, fusion tables, scripts, and other formats can be

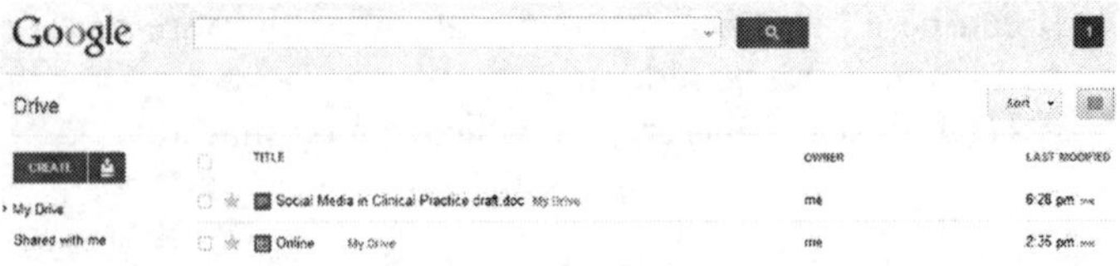

FIGURE 8.4 The dashboard of a Google Drive account with the documents assigned to the account (Google and the Google logo are registered trademarks of Google Inc., used with permission)

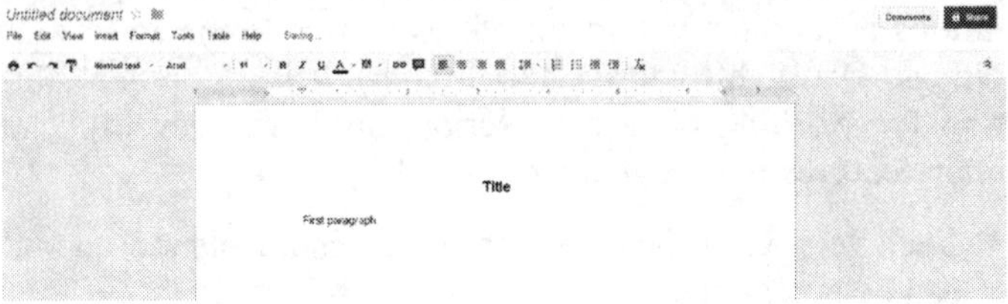

FIGURE 8.5 A new document on Google Docs (Google and the Google logo are registered trademarks of Google Inc., used with permission)

created if, in the latter case, the needed apps are downloaded. Creating a new document leads to an editing platform similar to those used in desktop based office softwares (Fig. 8.5).

In the document, a title can be added in the upper left corner, and comments can be assigned by using the button in the upper right corner. Versions are stored automatically by Google Docs. All the previous versions including the edits and the editor who made them can be accessed by File – See revision history. Document can be reverted to any previous versions.

New documents are created as private files which can only be accessed by the owner, but it can be shared by using the "Share" button in the upper right corner. The link of the document can be shared through social networking sites such as Google+, Facebook or Twitter; as well as with Google Mail contacts. All the users having any kind of access to the document (can edit, can comment or can only see) are listed here (Fig. 8.6).

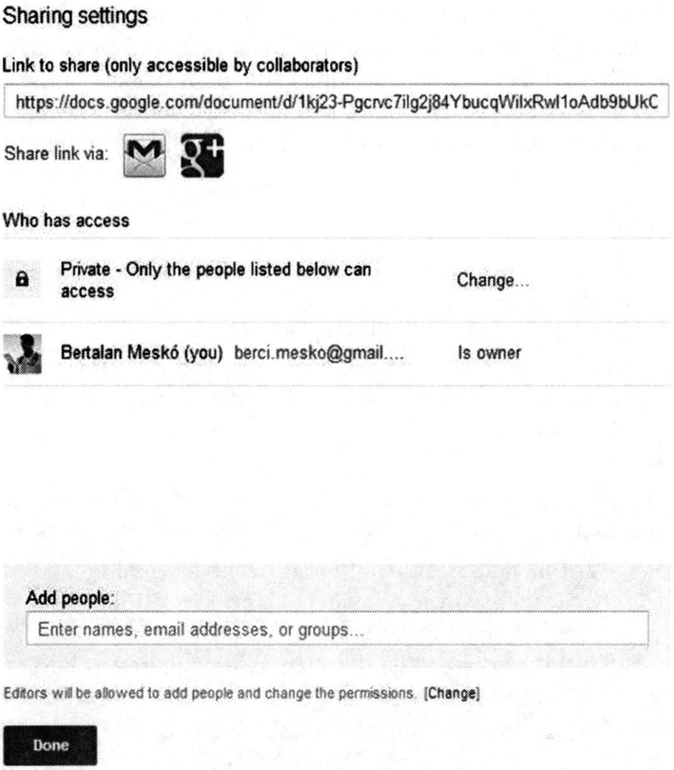

Sharing settings

Link to share (only accessible by collaborators)

https://docs.google.com/document/d/1kj23-Pgcrvc7ilg2j84YbucqWilxRwl1oAdb9bUkC

Share link via: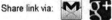

Who has access

🔒 Private - Only the people listed below can access   Change...

 Bertalan Meskó (you) berci.mesko@gmail....   Is owner

Add people:

Enter names, email addresses, or groups...

Editors will be allowed to add people and change the permissions. [Change]

Done

FIGURE 8.6 The share settings of a particular Google document (Google and the Google logo are registered trademarks of Google Inc., used with permission)

Zoho (http://www.zoho.com) or Conceptboard (http://www.conceptboard.com) can serve as an alternative to Google Docs.

Self-Test

1. Is it possible to edit a manuscript simultaneously online? Users can edit documents at the same time without interfering on Google Drive.

2. Which services are suitable for live group discussions?
   Examples include Skype, Google Hangout and FaceTalk.
3. What kind of documents can be edited on Google Docs?
   Documents, presentations, spreadsheets, forms, drawings,
   folders, fusion tables, scripts, and other formats as well.

Next Steps

1. Describe exactly what features are needed during the collaboration.
2. Find the services that suit your needs best.
3. Advise your colleagues and peers about using that particular service efficiently and enjoy the power of online collaboration.

Key Points

- Writing manuscripts, initiating group discussions and performing project management are all possible through online collaboration.
- Find the tool or service that suits your needs best and learn to use it.
- Choose the tools for online collaboration with a special focus on features, privacy and efficiency.

References

1. Alsharo M, Gregg D. Intention to collaborate: investigating online collaboration in virtual teams. AMCIS 2012 Proceedings. Paper 22. 2012.
2. Hyman JL, et al. Online professional networks for physicians: risk management. Clin Orthop Relat Res. 2012;470(5):1386–92.
3. Armfield NR, et al. Clinical use of Skype: a review of the evidence base. J Telemed Telecare. 2012;18(3):125–7.
4. Kippenbrock T, et al. Google docs: a better method than a paper clinical schedule. Comput Inform Nurs. 2010;28(3):138–40.

Chapter 9
Wikipedia and Medical Wikis

A wiki is a web page or collection of web pages designed to enable anyone with access to that to contribute to or modify its content via a web browser using a simplified markup language. Wikis are powered by wiki softwares. Wikis serve as platforms for online collaboration, knowledge management and notetaking [1]. Entries can be created, edited or deleted, as well as categories, templates or pages.

Ward Cunningham developed the first wiki software, WikiWikiWeb, as "the simplest online database that could possibly work" [2]. The word wiki is a Hawaiian word meaning "fast" or "quick". An important aspect of using wikis is the way the entries are inter-connected creating a simple way of collaboration.

Basic definitions used in wikis:

- edit allows the modification of the entries
- discussion or talk allows leaving comments for the entries on a different page
- history shows page history with all the previous edits with assigned times and dates; edit summaries and authors
- entry is a page in the wiki
- reversion makes it possible to substitute the current version of an entry with a previous one

Keywords and edit format of the wiki markup language: (Table 9.1)

B. Meskó, *Social Media in Clinical Practice*,
DOI 10.1007/978-1-4471-4306-2_9,
© Springer-Verlag London 2013

TABLE 9.1 Examples of the wiki markup language

The syntax language	What it looks like in the wiki
'''bold tex'''	**bold text**
[[medicine]]	medicine links to the entry about medicine
*unordered list	• unordered list
''italic formatting''	*italic formatting*
[http://www.page.com website]	website is a link to http://www.page.com

Wiki Platforms and Medical Ones

MediaWiki that powers Wikipedia can be installed on websites (http://www.mediawiki.org). This is one of the most popular wikis and a free open source package. Other alternatives include Wikispaces (http://www.wikispaces.com/) and Wikia (http://www.wikia.com). Anyone can create free wikis in order to facilitate online collaboration.

Medical professionals and organizations have been using wikis for creating a collaborative space in different specialties or around different topics. Generally only medical professionals providing credentials or copy of diploma can get access to these (Table 9.2).

Medpedia (http://www.medpedia.com/), an open platform for connecting people and information in order to advance medicine, was launched in co-operation with a group of medical schools as the medical alternative of Wikipedia [3].

A wiki's quality can be assessed based on different features:

- whether author or creator is described
- contact information is available
- the wiki is regularly updated
- whether categories are clear and well-thought
- medical content contributed by medical professionals is clearly separated from users without registration
- medical disclaimer is available

TABLE 9.2 Examples of medical wikis

Name of the wiki	URL of the wiki	Topic it focuses on
Askdrwiki	http://askdrwiki.com	Medical specialties
Radiopaedia	http://radiopaedia.org/	Radiology
HLwiki	http://hlwiki.slais.ubc.ca/	Medical librarianship
Ganfyd	http://www.ganfyd.org	Medicine
FluWikie	http://www.fluwikie.com/	Flu
WikiCancer	http://www.wikicancer.org/	Cancer
Clinfowiki	http://www.informatics-review.com	Clinical informatics
WikiKidney	http://www.wikikidney.org	Nephrology

Wikipedia, the Most Popular Wiki

Wikipedia (http://en.wikipedia.org) is without doubt the most popular wiki worldwide. This is a free, collaboratively edited, multilingual, online encyclopaedia launched in 2001 as a complementary project for Nupedia which was edited only by experts. It is supported by the non-profit Wikimedia Foundation. The basic idea was to create an encyclopaedia with the help of experts and non-experts by forming an online community with its own rules. By 2010, 53 % of American adult Internet users turned to Wikipedia [4].

The different roles of users in Wikipedia are defined by the community through polls [5]:

- steward: can grant or revoke any permission to or from any user on any wiki operated by the Wikimedia Foundation
- bureaucrat: can give administrator and bot rights
- administrator: can delete or protect pages, block or unblock users, among others.
- registered user: can edit and create entries
- unregistered user: can edit but not create new entries

The community of Wikipedia has defined rules, policies and guidelines for editing the entries and creating categories. The most important ones include:

- Entries are encyclopaedic and should represent a neutral point of view.
- Vandalism is not tolerated.
- Users should assume good faith and help new users.
- No original research should be added.
- Sources must be cited properly.
- Copyright violations must be avoided.
- New users are encouraged to make edits without asking for permission.

Vandalism is not uncommon in Wikipedia therefore the community makes sure false edits are reverted and factual errors are removed. Huggle is a software that facilitates this process with an easy to use interface [6].

The license of the content of Wikipedia was changed from GFDL to Creative Commons Attribution ShareAlike (CC BY-SA) 3.0. It means anyone is free to share, remix the content or make commercial use of it if attribution is given and the same license is used.

The quality of Wikipedia entries is assessed using different categories that help editors balance editorial focus.

- Featured articles represent the best content of Wikipedia.
- A class articles are close to be nominated as featured articles.
- Good articles are stable, well-written, referenced and show neutral point of view.
- B class
- C class
- Start class
- Stub: Only a few words.

The Wikimedia Foundation supports other projects as well (Table 9.3):

TABLE 9.3 The sister projects of Wikipedia

Name	URL	Basic description
Wiktionary	http://www.wiktionary.org/	Free dictionary
Wikibooks	http://www.wikibooks.org/	Open content textbooks
Wikiversity	http://www.wikiversity.org/	Open learning communities
Wikinews	http://www.wikinews.org/	News service
Wikispecies	http://species.wikimedia.org	Species directory
WikiMedia Commons	http://commons.wikimedia.org	Media library
Wikiquote	http://www.wikiquote.org/	Collection of quotations
Wikisource	http://wikisource.org	Free library

Collaborative Efforts in Medicine and Healthcare

There are several examples when medical organizations initiated collaborative efforts with Wikipedia. The National Institute of Health published guidelines about editing medical Wikipedia entries [7]. The scientific journal RNA Biology published guidelines that authors must submit a Wikipedia entry about their research on RNA families before submitting manuscripts to the journal [8]. Google and Wikipedia started a collaboration in which Google offered to hire experts who review medical and scientific entries [9].

Wikipedia can be a key tool in global public health promotion as both patients and medical professionals access information on that [10]. Moreover, a study concluded that cancer information found on Wikipedia was similar in accuracy and

TABLE 9.4 The medical projects of Wikipedia

Name of the project	URL	Description
WikiProject Medicine	http://en.wikipedia.org/wiki/Wikipedia:WikiProject_Medicine	A group that collaborates to improve the quality of Wikipedia's medicine and health-related articles
Portal Medicine	http://en.wikipedia.org/wiki/Portal:Medicine	Introduces the reader to key articles, images, and categories that further describe the subject and its related topics
Assessment	http://en.wikipedia.org/wiki/Wikipedia:WikiProject_Medicine/Assessment	Describes the quality and importance of medical Wikipedia entries
Collaboration of the month	http://en.wikipedia.org/wiki/Wikipedia:WikiProject_Medicine/Collaboration_of_the_Month	An entry is selected by polls every month which stays in focus by users

depth to the information on a peer-reviewed, patient-oriented cancer web site, but the readability of the information was questionable [11].

Medical projects are available for users who want to participate in the development of medical entries of Wikipedia. Main examples of medical Wikipedia projects are summarized in Table 9.4.

Self-Test

1. What kind of wiki platforms are available?
   Examples include MediaWiki, WikiSpaces and Wikia.
2. What kind of medical projects does Wikipedia have?
   WikiProject Medicine, Medicine Portal, and Collaboration of the month, among others.

3. Should a doctor edit a medical wiki or a medical entry on Wikipedia?

    It depends on the priorities of the doctor, the privacy settings of the wiki and whether the topic is for a broader audience.

Next Steps

1. Register by using a real name; create a profile with proper affiliation.
2. The Community Portal (http://en.wikipedia.org/wiki/Wikipedia:Community_portal) is a good starting point.
3. Portal:Medicine should help find the articles and categories of interest.
4. WikiProject Medicine invites users to sign up and look for projects they are open to work on.

When doing research online, a Wikipedia entry is a good place to start as it gives a clear picture of a particular topic, but should never be the last resource to finish the research with.

Key Points
- A wiki is a web page enabling anyone with access to that to contribute to its content using a simplified markup language.
- Medical wikis require credentials upon registration.
- Wikipedia is the most popular wiki that anyone can edit.
- Medical organizations and professionals initiated collaborative efforts with Wikipedia.
- When doing research online, a Wikipedia entry is a good place to start as it gives a clear picture of a particular topic, but should never be the last resource to finish the research with.

References

1. Wiki on Wikipedia. http://en.wikipedia.org/wiki/Wiki. Accessed 28 Jan 2013.
2. What Is Wiki. http://www.wiki.org/wiki.cgi?WhatIsWiki. Accessed 28 Jan 2013.
3. Rethlefsen MLS. Medpedia. J Med Libr Assoc. 2009;97(4):325–6.
4. 53 percent of online Americans use Wikipedia. http://pewinternet. org/Media-Mentions/2011/msnbc-Wikipedia.aspx. Accessed 28 Jan 2013.
5. Wikipedia:User access levels. http://en.wikipedia.org/wiki/ Wikipedia:User_access_levels. Accessed 28 Jan 2013.
6. Wikipedia:Huggle. http://en.wikipedia.org/wiki/Wikipedia:Huggle. Accessed 28 Jan 2013.
7. Guidelines for Participating in Wikipedia from NIH. http://www.nih. gov/icd/od/ocpl/resources/wikipedia/. Accessed 28 Jan 2013.
8. RNA Biology, Editorial Policies. http://www.landesbioscience.com/ journals/rnabiology/guidelines/. Accessed 28 Jan 2013.
9. Announcement to WikiProject Medicine community prior to trial editorial review. http://en.wikipedia.org/wiki/Wikipedia_ talk:WikiProject_Medicine/Archive_18#Announcement_to_ WikiProject_Medicine_community_prior_to_trial_editorial_review. Accessed 28 Jan 2013.
10. Heilman JM, et al. Wikipedia: a Key tool for global public health promotion. J Med Internet Res. 2011;13(1):e14.
11. Cancer Information On Wikipedia Is Accurate, But Not Very Readable. http://www.medicalnewstoday.com/releases/190536.php. Accessed 28 Jan 2013.

Chapter 10
Organizing Medical Events in Virtual Environments

Virtual environments have been used in cases when geographical limitations did not make real world meetings possible; when cost effective forms of communication or collaboration are needed or conferences have to be recorded, accessible online and archived. The combination of a community, learning materials, simulations and methods for communication can add up as a virtual environment. Virtual reality (VR) is a term applying to computer-simulated environments that can simulate physical presence in places in the real world, as well as in imaginary worlds [1]. Moreover, the number of virtual worlds has been increasing for the past few years [2].

One of the most popular virtual worlds is Second Life (http://www.secondlife.com) that was launched in 2003 and has over 20 million users [3]. In Second Life, users are represented as avatars and use different methods for communication. Users can explore virtual islands, build three dimensional objects, trade virtual property, socialize with other users or create educational materials. The virtual world is accessible by using a client software (Fig. 10.1).

The steps of entering Second Life:

1. Click on "Join now for free" on Secondlife.com
2. Choose an avatar
3. Choose a username (in order to participate in medical events it is advised to use a real name)
4. E-mail address, password, date of birth and security question/answer are needed.

B. Meskó, *Social Media in Clinical Practice*,
DOI 10.1007/978-1-4471-4306-2_10,
© Springer-Verlag London 2013

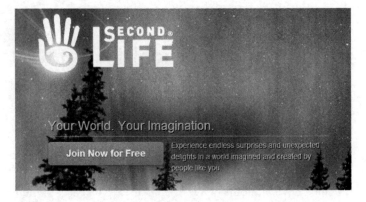

FIGURE 10.1 The main page of Second Life

5. Users have to choose between free and premium account (the latter one offers an own virtual house, virtual currency awards and gifts)
6. Download the software and install it.
7. Log in by using the username and password.

Orientation island gives a glimpse of the locations and content that can be accessed in-world such as music, social places, roleplaying, editors' pick or the most popular places (Fig. 10.2).

For medical professionals participating in projects in Second Life, the use of a real name and an appropriate avatar are recommended. Users can fly, walk, or use vehicles for moving around, although the most convenient way of moving is teleportation which means the user can be taken to any location if the exact co-ordinates are given.

The different ways of communication in Second Life are summarized in Table 10.1.

Examples of Using Second Life in Medicine

#1 Ann Myers Medical Center: A virtual education center that was launched in 2006. Conferences have been organized there, virtual case presentations have been presented as media content such as microscopic images, blood counts,

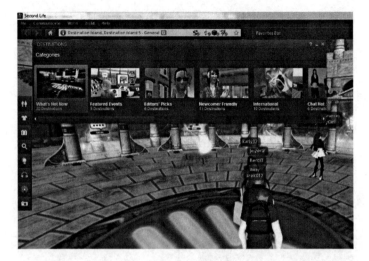

FIGURE 10.2 The opening area after logging into Second Life for the first time

TABLE 10.1 Ways of communication in Second Life

Way of communication	Details
Chat box	Avatars around can join the discussion
Instant messaging	Messages can be sent privately to users in-world
Voice chat	Avatars around can join the discussion
E-mail	Messages can be sent to avatars who are currently not in-world

radiology images can be uploaded, avatars can listen to cardiac and lung sounds, as well as perform basic procedures (e.g. intubation) [4] (Fig. 10.3).

#2 Heart Murmur Sim: Different rooms offer different virtual patients where avatars can listen to cardiac sounds and the task is to identify the proper diagnosis [5].

#3 SciFoo Lives On: A real world conference lived on in Second Life through posters and live presentations. The slideshows are hosted on the island of Nature Publishing Group [6].

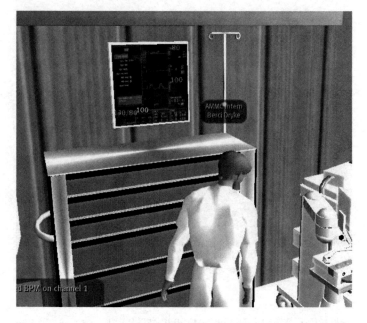

FIGURE 10.3 An avatar in a virtual clinical setting during a simulation

#4 Genome Island: A US teacher created an environment of an educational center focusing on genetics and genomics with 3D models, games and descriptions [7].

#5 Healthinfo Island: Educational materials are exhibited as posters for patients about different medical conditions and support centers with real staff are also available [8].

Organizing an Event in Second Life

It is possible to organize virtual meetings, presentations or exhibitions in Second Life which require a few steps.

1. A virtual location is needed (usually large medical organizations are open to land a place on their own island for such events).
2. Boards on which presentations can be presented should be installed. Presentations can be uploaded as image files or PDF.

3. The teleport link of the location is needed for the announcement.
4. A moderator is needed to control the event. In case voice chat does not work properly, it is advised to prepare texts in advance.

Second Life Alternatives

Second Life received criticism about the need for hardware and technical skills in order to be able to use for meetings or collaboration, therefore other platforms with simpler registration process were supported. Visuland (http://www.visuland.com) is a virtual environment which allows users to log in to a specific location within approximately 30 seconds. It was designed to avoid the technical problems associated with Second Life but it has much less users and activities.

Self-Test

1. What is the most popular virtual world?
   Second Life.
2. Is there a less technically challenging alternative to Second Life?
   Examples include Visuland.
3. What medical projects are there in Second Life?
   Users can listen to cardiac sounds; give or listen to presentations and present medical cases, among others.

Key Points
- Virtual environments have been used in cases when geographical limitations did not make real world meetings possible.
- The most popular virtual world is provided by Second Life.
- Several examples underscore the potential use of virtual worlds in medical education and patient groups.

References

1. Virtual Reality on Wikipedia. http://en.wikipedia.org/wiki/Virtual_reality. Accessed 28 Jan 2013.
2. Growth Forecasts for the Virtual Worlds Sector. http://www.kzero.co.uk/blog/?p=2845. Accessed 28 Jan 2013.
3. Second Life on Wikipedia. http://en.wikipedia.org/wiki/Second_Life. Accessed 28 Jan 2013.
4. The Ann Myers Medical Center. http://ammc.wordpress.com/. Accessed 28 Jan 2013.
5. Heart Murmur SIM. http://slhealthy.wetpaint.com/page/Heart+Murmur+SIM. Accessed 28 Jan 2013.
6. SciFoo Lives On Sessions. http://network.nature.com/groups/Second_Life/forum/topics/378. Accessed 28 Jan 2013
7. Genome Island. http://secondlife.com/destination/genome-island. Accessed 28 Jan 2013.
8. Health & Medicine in Second Life. http://healthinfoisland.blogspot.com. Accessed 28 Jan 2013.

Chapter 11
Medical Smartphone and Tablet Applications

There are approximately four billion mobile phones in the world, out of which 1.08 billion are smartphones. It is estimated that mobile Internet should take over desktop Internet usage by 2014 [1]. In 2012, 31 % of cell phone users used their phone to look for health information in the US, while this number was 17 % in 2010 [2].

The era of smartphones which are mobile phones built on a mobile operating system with advanced computing capability and connectivity, brought new opportunities in mobile health. The main smartphone operating systems include Google's Android, Apple's iOS, Nokia's Symbian, RIM's BlackBerry OS, Samsung's Bada, Microsoft's Windows Phone, Hewlett-Packard's webOS and embedded Linux.

Mobile health or mHealth can be defined as the delivery of healthcare services via mobile communication devices [3]. As mobile Internet access becomes a globally recognizable trend, it is inevitable to see more and more mHealth initiatives. It can include the usage of text message (SMS), smartphone applications or home monitoring devices.

Main Differences Among Mobile Operating Systems

As users have different needs about a mobile device, the comparison of features might help choose the hardware and software that suit our needs best [4] (Table 11.1).

B. Meskó, *Social Media in Clinical Practice*,
DOI 10.1007/978-1-4471-4306-2_11,
© Springer-Verlag London 2013

TABLE 11.1 Differences between mobile operating systems

	Android	**iOS**	**Windows Phone**
Company	Google	Apple	Microsoft
License	Free and open-source	end-user license agreement	Proprietary
Browser search engine options	Many	Bing, Google, Yahoo Search	Bing, Google
Multitasking	Yes	Limited	Yes
Cost of developing apps	Free ($25 once to offer it on the Google Play)	Free ($99/year to distribute on App Store)	Free ($99/year to offer it on the Windows Phone Store)

TABLE 11.2 Resources and databases of medical smartphone applications

Name	**URL**	**Short description**
Webicina	http://www.webicina.com	Curated medical smartphone apps focusing on specialties and conditions
iMedicalApps	http://www.imedicalapps.com/	Blog publishing reviews of medical apps
Appolicious	http://www.appolicious.com/categories/26-health-fitness	Database of iOS apps in health and fitness
AppBrain	http://www.appbrain.com/apps/highest-rated/medical/	Database of Android medical apps

Medical Smartphone Applications

Smartphone apps are applications users run on smartphones. The number of medical and health-related iOS, Android and Windows Phone smartphone apps in the iOS App Store, Google Play and Windows App Store, respectively has been increasing for years. Searching for relevant apps requires properly designed and managed databases (Table 11.2).

Features to be checked before choosing a smartphone application:

- Check the author of the app, is it a real entity?
- Check out the reviews/ratings whether those are mostly positive.
- Check out comments looking for feedback.
- The app should be updated regularly. The publication date of the latest version is always shown.
- Choose apps that were designed for the mobile operating system of interest.
- Screenshots and videos assigned to the app profiles can also be helpful.

Medical or health-related smartphone apps can be divided into two main categories such as apps for consumers, and medical professionals.

Smartphone Apps for Consumers

Consumers use apps for their own health management, for keeping in touch with their doctors or for other health-related reasons. Real examples might represent the main ways of using smartphone apps as patients.

Example #1: Sensors or devices that measure health parameters such as blood sugar content can be attached to smartphones associated with a relevant smartphone app that logs and visualizes the levels. Results can be shared with the doctor.

Example #2: Augmented reality is a live view of the real-world environment augmented by computer-generated sensory input such as sound, video, graphics or GPS data. It means looking through a mobile phone's camera yields additional information from e.g. online resources. Apps can be developed that makes it possible for people with color blindness to see real colors [5].

Example #3: The Dutch university UMC Utrecht launched a project under the name Telebaby in which cameras were installed at the incubators of pediatrics departments and

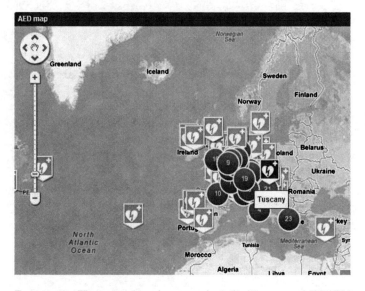

FIGURE 11.1 The map of semi-automatic defibrillators on AED4EU

parents could watch their children live 24 h a day through a mobile device [6].

Example #4: UMC St Radboud in the Netherlands launched AED4.eu in 2009 with the ambition to map all automatic electronic defibrillators in the Netherlands which can be accessed via augmented reality by using a mobile phone. As of 2013, it covers several countries [7] (Fig. 11.1).

Smartphone Apps for Medical Professionals

All stakeholders of healthcare use smartphone apps either for personal or professional reasons. The challenges of using apps during work include regulations related to the Health Insurance Accountability and Portability Act which was inacted in order to protect the privacy of patients; whether the apps and the electronic medical record system of the healthcare institution are inter-connected or compatible; and whether the institution's policy approves the use of smartphones during work hours.

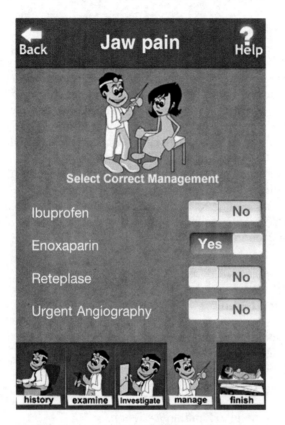

FIGURE 11.2 The main page of the Prognosis application

Example #1: The iCard ECG application for iOS devices can record 30 s of the patient's heart's rhythmic pulse and perform heart monitoring [8]. The AliveCor device was approved by the FDA to measure ECG with a smartphone [9].

Example #2: Pocketbody brings three dimensional anatomical structures to iOS devices [10].

Example #3: Prognosis published medical case studies in numerous medical specialties on different mobile operating systems (http://www.prognosisapp.com/) (Fig. 11.2).

Example #4: A Swedish dermatology practice developed an Android and iPhone application through which patients can submit photos of their skin condition which is analyzed for a fee (http://idoc24.com).

Tablets in Medicine

A tablet is a mobile computer operated by touchscreen on which the user's finger functions as the mouse and cursor. Introducing tablets into medicine and healthcare brought new possibilities as the larger screen and the easier navigation make them potentially useful for medical usage. Based on a 2012 survey, 62 % of physicians owned a tablet computer; and half of them use it at the point of care [11].

Tablets are used at several medical schools in education; in operating rooms, as well as in medical imaging [12].

The assessment of the quality of tablet-based medical apps is based on the same features that were described in relation to smartphone apps.

Potential Uses of Mobile Technology in Healthcare

- Appointment and medication reminders by SMS
- Patient support by SMS
- Accessing electronic patient records
- Smart homes in elderly care
- Patient diaries for clinical trials
- Locating blood and organ donors
- Patient consent
- Linking emergency services
- Disease monitoring
- Food and environmental contamination alerts
- Wireless stethoscope and other medical devices

Self-Test

1. What is a smartphone?
   A mobile phone built on a mobile operating system with advanced computing capability and connectivity.
2. What features should be checked before choosing a medical smartphone application?

The author, reviews, ratings, and updates, among others.
3. What is the difference between a tablet and a smartphone? A tablet is a mobile computer operated by touchscreen on which the user's finger functions as the mouse and cursor.

Key Points
- Mobile health or mHealth can be defined as the delivery of healthcare services via mobile communication devices.
- The era of smartphones brought new opportunities in mobile health.
- The quality of medical smartphone apps should be assessed by medical professionals who can "prescribe" apps for their patients.
- Tablets are used at several medical schools in education; in operating rooms, as well as in medical imaging.
- Using mobile technologies is now part of the practice of medicine.

References

1. Infographic: Are you paying attention to #mhealth?. http://www.healthcarecommunication.com/Main/Articles/7468.aspx. Accessed 28 Jan 2013.
2. Mobile Health 2012. http://www.pewinternet.org/Reports/2012/Mobile-Health.aspx. Accessed 28 Jan 2013.
3. The mHealth Summit: Local & Global Converge. http://www.caroltorgan.com/mhealth-summit/. Accessed 28 Jan 2013.
4. Comparison of mobile operating systems on Wikipedia. http://en.wikipedia.org/wiki/Comparison_of_mobile_operating_systems. Accessed 28 Jan 2013.
5. DanKam smartphone app aids the color-blind. http://news.cnet.com/8301-27080_3-20026054-245.html. Accessed 28 Jan 2013.
6. Telebaby. http://www.umcutrecht.nl/subsite/Telebaby/. Accessed 28 Jan 2013.
7. aed4.eu. http://www.aed4.eu/?language=en. Accessed 28 Jan 2013.

8. iCard ECG brings heart monitoring to the iOS device of your choice (video).   http://www.engadget.com/2011/06/20/icard-ecg-brings-heart-monitoring-to-the-ios-device-of-your-choi/. Accessed 28 Jan 2013.

9. Pocket Anatomy. https://itunes.apple.com/us/app/pocket-body/id388633565?mt=8. Accessed 28 Jan 2013.

10. Mobile Health Moves Forward: FDA Approves AliveCor's Heart Monitor For The iPhone. http://techcrunch.com/2012/12/04/mobile-health-moves-forward-fda-approves-alivecors-heart-monitor-for-the-iphone/. Accessed 26 Mar 2013.

11. Doctors quick to adopt tablets into practice. http://www.ama-assn.org/amednews/2012/06/04/bil20604.htm. Accessed 28 Jan 2013.

12. iPads In Health And Medicine: More Than An Information Revolution? http://www.medicalnewstoday.com/articles/242843.php. Accessed 28 Jan 2013.

Chapter 12
Use of Social Media by Hospitals and Medical Practices

Health 2.0 is a term referring to the interaction between healthcare institutions and medical practices; and social media [1]. As social media is becoming more popular among e-patients, it was a clear trend that hospitals and medical practices would start using it for creating an online presence and keeping in touch with patients.

A few examples what purposes hospitals can use social media channels for:

1. **Customer service**: replying to messages coming from non-traditional resources in a fast and accurate way (Fig. 12.1).
2. **Community outreach**: social media provides solutions with which people living in the proximity of the hospital can be targeted with messages and announcements. It can also play a major role in crisis communication.
3. **Patient education**: the online presence of hospitals gives opportunity for reaching patients in a widespread way and educate them about health issues, prevention or healthy lifestyle. Mayo Clinic launched a campaign "Know Your Numbers" in 2012 about the importance of knowing the number of health parameters such as blood pressure or body mass index. Patients could calculate their risk for heart disease with a Facebook application and earn points by spreading the word about the campaign through social media [2].

B. Meskó, *Social Media in Clinical Practice*, 109
DOI 10.1007/978-1-4471-4306-2_12,
© Springer-Verlag London 2013

> @ChildrensPgh hi, I am due to start a
> project on child palliative care, do u
> have any info or stats I could use? I can
> provide an e-mail :)
> Nurse_Mikey (Mikey Whitehead)

> @Nurse_Mikey sure, give me an e-mail
> and I could connect you with someone
> who might be able to help.
> ChildrensPgh (Children's Hospital)

FIGURE 12.1 Twitter messages exchanged between a nurse and a hospital

4. **Real-time experience**: Certain hospitals have experienced with streaming operations live via social media channels such as Twitter or Instagram [3, 4].
5. **Improving public relations (PR)**: Social media channels allow hospitals to create an online presence and improve the company profile. Such presence includes the announcement of milestones, research results, current events, community news or renovations.

Adoption Curve of Social Media

Hospitals embracing social media needs to take certain steps that include observation of what similar resources communicate online; education of their target audience with their own content; broadcasting messages and announcements; participating in online discussions and projects; making relationships with their audience; and finally real collaboration with patients to improve their care (Fig. 12.2).

Data underscore the use of social media by hospitals as the social media accounts of over a 1,000 hospitals are included in a constantly updated database [5].

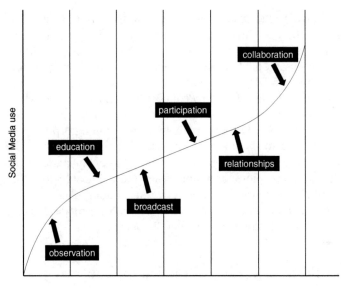

FIGURE 12.2 Hospitals' adoption curve of social media

A Successful Social Media Presence by Mayo Clinic

Mayo Clinic (http://www.mayoclinic.com/) has been leading the health 2.0 movement by creating an example of using social media properly. Accounts Mayo Clinic has been managing:

- Youtube channel where patient interviews are published (http://www.youtube.com/user/mayoclinic).
- Twitter channel for posting news and announcements (https://twitter.com/MayoClinic).
- Facebook page for keeping in touch with patients (http://www.facebook.com/MayoClinic).
- Blog serving as a communication channel (http://www.mayoclinic.org/blogs/).

Mayo Clinic also launched the Mayo Clinic Center for Social Media (http://socialmedia.mayoclinic.org/), a media center focused on healthcare using the leadership of Mayo Clinic among healthcare providers in adopting social media resources. In 2011, a patient community was launched under the name "Connect" (http://connect.mayoclinic.org/) on which visitors can upload photos, watch health videos and stories from patients, meet other patients with a shared purpose.

In order to show a potential benefit of using social media with strategy, Mayo Clinic ran a pilot study giving patients the option to complete an online structured medical history that would be reviewed by a doctor within 24 hours. According to their estimations, the online consultations made surgery appointments unnecessary in 40 % of cases [6].

Building a Medical Practice Online

Social media can provide a good way for building an online presence for a medical practice and finding its target audience but only if it is used properly with a clear strategy. The design and development of such a strategy requires specific steps.

1. **Observation**: Medical professionals in many areas are already online and publish content on certain social media channels. Listening to them and observing the communication they use is advised before launching any channels.
2. **Designing a social media strategy**: The goals must be defined in details and a plan about evaluating the results from time to time is much needed.
3. **Designing a social media policy**: It must be stated in a clear way what a medical professional can communicate and how patients can communicate with them through these online channels. Some rules are written such as those of the American Medical Association [7]; other rules represent the common sense such as not writing things online which the author would never say in the offline world.
4. **An own website**: Although social media channels can take up the majority of communication, an own website is still needed for representing the official channel of the company

TABLE 12.1 How social media platforms can be used in healthcare

Social media platform	Uniqueness
Twitter	Rapid discussions, but no longer descriptions
Facebook	Community building, but less customization
Blog (e.g. Wordpress, Blogger)	Serving as an online CV and communication channel
Youtube	Recommended place for uploading videos
Flickr	Photo collections

containing links to the social channels as well. It should have a clear interface with a simple design, detailed description of the practice; author information and credentials with full names. Dynamic updates in the content with an easily accessible RSS feed are recommended.

5. **Choosing the appropriate social media channels**: Based on the above mentioned points, one can choose the right channels, normally, one or two which should be updated regularly. Different social media platforms bear with different advantages (Table 12.1).

The potential benefits of using social media properly for managing a medical practice:

- Increasing patient traffic.
- Being up-to-date by following and communicating with peers.
- Acting as a filter online for the patients leads to building trust before the first meeting.
- As patients do searches for the name of their doctor online, it is important to control the information being published about us.

Self-Test

1. What purposes can hospitals use social media channels for?
   Customer service, community outreach, patient education, real time experience and improving PR.
2. What was launched by Mayo Clinic to lead the adoption of social media resources?
   Mayo Clinic Center for Social Media.

3. What are the main steps of building a medical practice online? Observation, designing a social media strategy and a policy, and choosing the appropriate social media channels.

Key Points
- Health 2.0 is a term referring to the interaction between healthcare institutions and medical practices and social media.
- Hospitals and medical practices use social media for creating an online presence and keeping in touch with patients.
- Mayo Clinic has been leading the health 2.0 movement by creating an example of using social media properly.
- Social media provides a good way for building an online presence for a medical practice but only with strategy.

References

1. Health 2.0 on Wikipedia. http://en.wikipedia.org/wiki/Health_2.0. Accessed 28 Jan 2013.
2. "Know Your Numbers" is National Anthem of Heart Month. http://newsblog.mayoclinic.org/2012/01/26/know-your-numbers-is-national-anthem-of-heart-month/. Accessed 20 June 2013.
3. World's First Live-Tweeted Open-Heart Surgery is a Success [PICS]. http://mashable.com/2012/02/23/tweeted-open-heart-surgery/. Accessed 28 Jan 2013.
4. Surgeons send 'tweets' from operating room. http://articles.cnn.com/2009-02-17/tech/twitter.surgery_1_twitter-and-facebook-social-networking-site-twitter-tweeted?_s=PM:TECH. Accessed 28 Jan 2013.
5. Health Care Social Media List. http://network.socialmedia.mayo-clinic.org/hcsml-grid/. Accessed 28 Jan 2013.
6. Mayo cuts appointments by 40 per cent. http://www.ehi.co.uk/news/primary-care/6259. Accessed 28 Jan 2013.
7. "New AMA Policy Helps Guide Physicians' Use of Social Media". http://www.ama-assn.org/ama/pub/news/news/social-media-policy.page. Accessed 28 Jan 2013.

Chapter 13
Medical Video and Podcast

Media content has been undergoing major changes in the past couple of years due to the changing nature of the Internet and the way consumers follow media channels. Media has been centered around video and audio content instead of text. This notion was further underscored when the Person of the Year award was given to "You", the users of Internet, by TIME magazine and the award was illustrated by an online video player as one of the most essential components of social media [1].

On the 23rd of April, 2005 the first video was uploaded on a new website designed for showing and collecting videos contributed by users. It was called Youtube which was acquired by Google in 2006 and went through several steps of development before becoming the most popular video browser in the world. The most popular video ever uploaded to Youtube has over 1.6 billion viewers as of June, 2013 [2] (Table 13.1).

Users can upload videos up to 15 min each in duration, but users with a good track record of complying with the site's Community Guidelines may upload videos up to 12 h in length. Youtube channels must be assigned to Google accounts which allow users to collect videos around a particular topic. In order to launch a Youtube channel, the creation of a new user account is advised. A Youtube channel with medical content should contain specific pieces of information:

- Full name of the author/curator
- Affiliation and location
- Proper name and description of the channel

B. Meskó, *Social Media in Clinical Practice*,
DOI 10.1007/978-1-4471-4306-2_13,
© Springer-Verlag London 2013

TABLE 13.1 Main developments and timeline of Youtube.com

Time	Main developments
2005	Official launch and the first video uploaded
2006	Acquisition by Google
2007	First High Definition (HD) channels
2009	First concert streamed live
2012–13	Over four billion videos streamed per day [3]

- Contact information
- A proper banner which can be placed on top of the channel with additional information about the practice, topic or institution.

Materials with copyright should not be uploaded and videos must always follow the community guidelines set by Youtube. An important information about uploaded videos is that users retain copyrights as stated in the Terms of Service [4]:

> For clarity, you retain all of your ownership rights in your Content. However, by submitting Content to YouTube, you hereby grant YouTube a worldwide, non-exclusive, royalty-free, sublicenseable and transferable license to use, reproduce, distribute, prepare derivative works of, display, and perform the Content in connection with the Service and YouTube's (and its successors' and affiliates') business, including without limitation for promoting and redistributing part or all of the Service (and derivative works thereof) in any media formats and through any media channels.

Good examples of medical Youtube channels give a hint about the creation of a new channel (Table 13.2).

The most viewed medical video has had over 160 million views as of February, 2013; and it is about the video stroboscopy of the vocal cords [5].

Reasons of getting closer to Youtube as a medical professional include the fact that Youtube is now the second largest

TABLE 13.2 Examples of medical Youtube channels

Youtube channel	URL	Topic
Fauquier ENT	http://www.youtube.com/user/fauquierent	Otolaryngology
HemOnc Today	http://www.youtube.com/user/HemOncToday	Hematology/oncology
Society of General Internal Medicine	http://www.youtube.com/user/TheSGIM	Internal Medicine
European Society of Cardiology	http://www.youtube.com/user/escardiodotorg	Cardiology
Dr Jerry Gordon	http://www.youtube.com/user/DrJerryGordon	Dentistry
Clinical Neurology News	http://www.youtube.com/user/ClinNeurologyNews	Neurology

search engine online [6]; a large number of medical video channels can be found there; doctors and patients have already been using it for medicine-related purposes [7].

Alternative Sites for Videos

There are other sites in which user generated video content can be uploaded and shared. Examples include Ustream (http://www.ustream.tv), Vimeo (http://vimeo.com/) and Justin.tv (http://www.justin.tv/). Ustream and Justin.tv also allow users to broadcast events or presentations live.

Medical Video Sites

Since the launch of Youtube, many other websites featuring video content but specifically in medicine and healthcare have appeared. Usually such websites have a proper medical disclaimer stating the education nature of the content instead of giving medical advice; clear privacy policy, site description

TABLE 13.3 Examples of medical video sites

Name	URL	Most important feature
Video, MD	http://www.videomd.com/	Focuses on physician-patient education
eMedTV	http://www.emedtv.com/	Videos for patients created by experts
The Doctor's Channel	http://www.thedoctorschannel.com/	Short videos for doctors
OR Live	http://www.orlive.com/	Online Surgical and Healthcare Video and Webcasts
SciVee TV	http://www.scivee.tv/	Videos describing biomedical research findings

and the fact that the videos are intended for medical professionals only. There are video sites for only medical professionals in peer-to-peer communication; for patient education and for self-learning (Table 13.3).

Videos created by medical professionals for any of the above mentioned reasons should be of good quality, contain only appropriate content and targeted for the specific audiences. Things to consider before uploading a video online include:

- whether the content of the video is appropriate
- whether it should be available in a public or in a private way (uploaded videos on Youtube can be marked as public or private which can only be seen by users getting access to that)
- whether patient information is removed from the video

Podcasts in Medicine and Healthcare

A podcast is a type of digital media consisting of an episodic series of files (either audio or video) subscribed to and downloaded through web syndication. Audio podcasts became popular as through them users can listen to articles, texts,

TABLE 13.4 Examples of medical podcasts

Name of the podcast	URL
The Journal of the American Medical Association	http://jama.jamanetwork.com/multimedia.aspx#Weekly
The New England Journal of Medicine Weekly Summary	http://www.nejm.org/multimedia/audio-summary
The Medical University of South Carolina	http://www.muschealth.com/multimedia/Podcasts
Annals of Internal Medicine Podcast	https://itunes.apple.com/us/podcast/annals-internal-medicine-podcast/id259716343
Johns Hopkins Medicine News Roundup	http://www.hopkinsmedicine.org/news/audio/podcasts/

posts or research findings via MP3 files or other format instead of reading those in front of the screen.

For this reason, numerous medical journals and organizations have embraced this technology and have been providing their followers with regular podcasts (Table 13.4).

Directories of medical podcasts are available online and constantly updated [8–10].

Creating and sharing quality podcasts featuring nonpersonal information about medical conditions with patients in a private way may save time for medical professionals as well as help build a relationship with the patient based on trust. Wendy Sue Swanson, MD publishes such materials in the form of podcasts or videos in order to educate her patients [11]; while Mike Sevilla, MD launched the first online medical radio show, the Dr. Anonymous Show which later was changed to Family Medicine Rocks creating a respected online presence for him [12].

Creating Podcasts

Several platforms enable users to create podcast channels such as BlogTalkRadio (http://www.blogtalkradio.com/), PodBean (http://www.podbean.com/) or PodOmatic (http://

www.podomatic.com). Otherwise recording can be performed with a simple audio recorder or even with Skype and the mp3 files can be shared.

Creating a channel usually requires the audio file, a title, short description and a category. It is advised to choose platforms on which podcasts can be accessed for free.

Communicating with the Media

The rise of social media led to larger exposure for medical professionals and as the members of traditional media such as reporters or newswriters also use these channels for gathering information, a few suggestions may facilitate building a proper relationship with them.

- Be open and available: reporters tend to choose interviewees who are easy to reach online.
- Do not underestimate their medical knowledge, instead try to assist them in their work with additional resources and pieces of information.
- Always make sure to see the final version before publication and use written discussions (e.g. archived e-mails) to prove your point later on if needed.
- Try to get questions or interest areas before an interview. It is a mutual goal to be prepared for an interview.

Self-Test

1. What information should a medical Youtube channel contain?
   Full name of the author/curator, affiliation and location; and contact information.
2. Who owns the rights of the uploaded videos on Youtube?
   Users retain all of the ownership rights in their content.
3. Why would a medical professional create a podcast?
   To share non-personal information about medical conditions with patients in a private way saving time and building a relationship with the patient.

Key Points
- Media content has been undergoing major changes due to the way consumers follow media channels.
- Youtube is the second largest search engine and features a large number of medical video channels.
- Websites featuring video content but specifically in medicine and healthcare have appeared.
- A podcast is a type of digital media consisting of a series of audio or video files subscribed to and downloaded through web syndication.

References

1. You (Time Person of the Year) on Wikipedia. http://en.wikipedia.org/wiki/You_(Time_Person_of_the_Year). Accessed 28 Jan 2013.
2. PSY - Gangnam Style. http://www.youtube.com/watch?v=9bZkp7q19f0&feature=share&list=LLinU1twr8pRPNJyIoizLAQA. Accessed 28 Jan 2013.
3. Exclusive: YouTube hits 4 billion daily video views. http://www.reuters.com/article/2012/01/23/us-google-youtube-idUSTRE80M0TS20120123. Accessed 28 Jan 2013.
4. Terms of Service of Youtube. http://www.youtube.com/static?template=terms. Accessed 28 Jan 2013.
5. Video Stroboscopy of the Vocal Cords (video). http://www.youtube.com/watch?v=ajbcJiYhFKY. Accessed 28 Jan 2013.
6. YouTube: The Monster Search Engine You Can't Ignore. http://www.mediapost.com/publications/article/163492/youtube-the-monster-search-engine-you-cant-ignor.html#axzz2IccWnpsl. Accessed 28 Jan 2013.
7. Doctors Using YouTube for Patient Education, Professional Networking. http://www.ihealthbeat.org/articles/2012/6/19/doctors-using-youtube-for-patient-education-professional-networking.aspx. Accessed 28 Jan 2013.
8. Medical Podcasts and Videocasts: List. https://spreadsheets.google.com/pub?key=p6MskqOaqmuB8_TNGgB_yOg. Accessed 28 Jan 2013.
9. Medical podcasts & videocasts on HLWiki Canada. http://hlwiki.slais.ubc.ca/index.php/Podcasts_and_Videocasts. Accessed 28 Jan 2013.
10. Podmedics Library. http://www.podmedics.com/library. Accessed 28 Jan 2013.
11. Seattle Mama Doc on Youtube. http://www.youtube.com/playlist?list=PLFDF0A4E130F59AEF&feature=plcp. Accessed 28 Jan 2013.
12. Family Medicine Rocks. http://www.familymedicinerocks.com/. Accessed 28 Jan 2013.

Chapter 14
Creating Presentations and Slideshows

Interpreting and sharing research results and clinical findings became more important than ever as social media is changing the landscape of online communication. The common way of doing that is by giving presentations online and offline. As clinicians are overwhelmed and being up-to-date is more challenging than ever, giving clear and engaging presentations is demanding.

A series of suggestions and pieces of advice might help improve presentations skills and materials.

- Use images wisely: Visual slides could transmit a message with more success than a whole slide of text. Quality images can be found in commercial, royalty free image databases such as Stockxpert (http://www.stockxpert.com/) or bigStockPhoto (http://www.bigstockphoto.com/).
- Talk instead of including all the texts you have in the slides: People read faster than you talk.
- Don't read your text neither from your slides, nor from a paper. It makes it impossible to create a connection with the audience.
- Personal stories make even research findings more appealing.
- Practice is the most important part of a presentation.
- Interruptions happen and speakers should be prepared for that.
- No matter how scientific the slideshow is, only passionate and prepared speakers can transmit the essential messages to the audience.

B. Meskó, *Social Media in Clinical Practice*, 123
DOI 10.1007/978-1-4471-4306-2_14,
© Springer-Verlag London 2013

- Each slide should be optimized regarding image quality, amount of text and the size of text according to the particular audience.
- Every audience is different requiring special preparation; experienced speaker should be able to adjust the way of presenting to the actual mood and focus of the audience during the talk.
- Speakers should value every question they receive and encourage the audience to ask more.

Avoiding Last Minute Surprises

Presenters might have to face technical problems before or during the presentation. A few tricks might be of help:

- Putting the presentation on a USB drive
- Saving the slideshow in PDF format as well to avoid compatibility problems regarding Powerpoint.
- Uploading the slideshow online (e.g. Google Drive – https://drive.google.com, or Dropbox – https://www.dropbox.com) for safety reasons.
- Use commonly known font styles such as Times New Roman.
- Be aware of the observation that some presenters do not show the margins properly therefore content can be hidden from the audience.
- In case of large presentation rooms, the use of larger fonts is advised.
- Screensaver, e-mail or virus alerts and notifications should be turned off during the presentation.

Methods for Giving a Presentation

Besides traditional methods, there are special ones that might be used even in scientific and medical events.

Lessig Method: Stanford Law professor Lawrence Lessig created his own method for giving slideshows as his slides often contained just a single word, short quote, or a photo and talks for only a few seconds per slide.

PechaKucha: A format which keeps the presentations concise and fast-paced, as only 20 slides are used and each slide is shown for 20 s (6 min and 40 s in total).

10/20/30: Guy Kawasaki promoted the 10/20/30 Rule of PowerPoint: "a PowerPoint presentation should have ten slides, last no more than 20 min, and contain no font smaller than 30 points" [1].

Tools and Platforms for Creating Presentations

There are several softwares and online platforms either for creating or giving a presentation out of which Powerpoint and Keynote are the most popular softwares, while Google Drive (https://drive.google.com) and Sliderocket (http://www.sliderocket.com) are available online. Prezi (http://www.prezi.com) allows the creation of presentations either online or with an offline editor and it provides a free educational account. Prezi lets users explore and share ideas on a virtual canvas (Table 14.1).

The similarities and differences between these services are shown based on the new presentation panel and the editor dashboard. After starting to create a new presentation, a template can be chosen in both services which helps the user start from sketches (Figs. 14.1 and 14.2).

The Prezi editor dashboard contains several features including the addition of frames, images, shapes, media content or a Powerpoint file. The frames can be connected to each

TABLE 14.1 Comparisons of presentation creator tools

Name	Creator	Main feature
Powerpoint	Microsoft	Most popular software
Keynote	Apple	A software with a tablet-based version as well
Prezi.com	Prezi	Cloud-based presentation software
Google Drive	Google	Web-based platform
Sliderocket.com	Sliderocket	Web-based platform

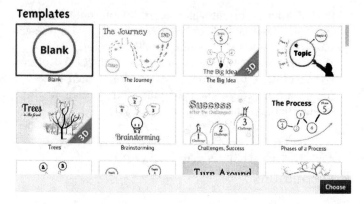

FIGURE 14.1 Templates offered by Prezi.com (Image is used with permission from Prezi.com)

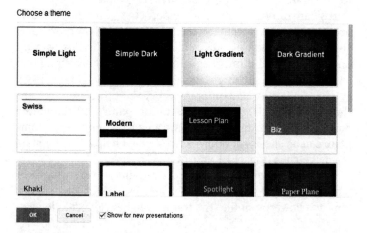

FIGURE 14.2 Templates offered by Google Docs (Google and the Google logo are registered trademarks of Google Inc., used with permission)

other by editing a path of slides; the editor can be shared with other authors through Prezi Meeting and the content can be edited by using a special zooming user interface (Fig. 14.3).

The Google Drive presentation editor is similar to the other editor formats of the service such as document or

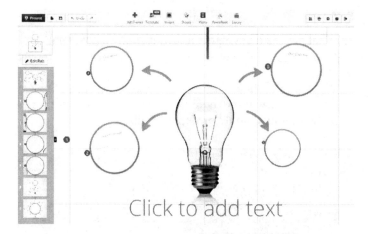

FIGURE 14.3 The editor dashboard after creating a new presentation on Prezi.com (Image is used with permission from Prezi.com)

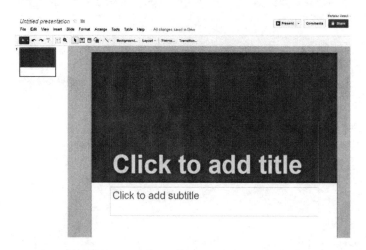

FIG. 14.4 A new presentation creating on Google Docs (Google and the Google logo are registered trademarks of Google Inc., used with permission)

spreadsheet editing. The slideshow can be shared easily with other co-authors or viewers as well (Fig. 14.4).

Self-Test

1. What are the main platforms for creating a presentation?
   Examples include Powerpoint, Keynote, Prezi and Google Docs.
2. What are the clinical aspects of creating a presentation?
   Patient information should be removed from slides and patient photos should be depersonalized.

Key Points
- Interpreting and sharing research results and clinical findings is crucial.
- Practice and other suggestions can help improve the quality of presentations.
- There are several tools for creating presentations and choosing the right platform requires efforts.

Reference

1. The 10/20/30 Rule of PowerPoint. http://blog.guykawasaki.com/2005/12/the_102030_rule.html. Accessed 28 Jan 2013.

Chapter 15
E-mails and Privacy Concerns

E-mail or electronic mail is a method of sending and receiving digital messages online. This is one of the most common forms of online communication and while patients usually send simple questions via e-mail to their doctors, it might contain sensitive information which could lead to legal consequences if medical professionals do not know about such potential issues and the ways to avoid these.

It is inevitable that patients would use that for asking medical advice, moreover the possibility of exchanging e-mails with their physicians led to a better overall patient satisfaction for patients [1].

Eighty-five percentage of patients stated e-mail would be a good way to communicate with their physicians [2]. The most common topics in patients' e-mails include [3]:

- Prescription refills
- Scheduling appointments
- Confirming appointments
- Test results
- Medical advice and request for additional health information
- Clarification of treatment plans
- Release of medical records

The potential advantages and disadvantages of using e-mails in the doctor-patient relationship (Table 15.1).

B. Meskó, *Social Media in Clinical Practice*,   129
DOI 10.1007/978-1-4471-4306-2_15,
© Springer-Verlag London 2013

TABLE 15.1 Potential advantages and disadvantages of using e-mails in medical communication

Advantages	Concerns
Inexpensive and rapid	Inappropriate use for certain medical conditions
Improve access to online educational materials	Potential for increased physician workload
Reduces the number of telephone calls	Legal issues
Increase patient participation in medical decision-making	Privacy problems

A typical e-mail consists of:

- From: The e-mail address and the name of the author who sends the e-mail.
- To: The e-mail address and optionally the name of the recipient who will receive the e-mail.
- Add Cc: The e-mail addresses and optionally the names of those who would get a copy of the e-mail.
- Add Bcc: The same as Cc but these e-mail addresses are hidden from the recipient.
- Subject line that defines the topic of the e-mail.
- Attach file: Different file types such as document or images can be attached to the e-mails.
- Text of the message which can contain videos, images or links to websites.
- Signature

As e-mail messages are not encrypted, go through intermediate networks before reaching the final destinations; and the e-mail addresses and names in the e-mail prevent anonymous communication, privacy concerns have been discussed in the literature. An example of a medical disclaimer that should be placed in the bottom of e-mails:

This e-mail and any files transmitted with it are confidential and intended solely for the use of the individual or entity to whom they are addressed. If you have received this e-mail in error please notify the system manager.

Information in this e-mail is intended for educational purposes only and does not replace the relationship that exists between a patient and his/her physician; and does not provide medical advice.

Suggestions About Dealing with E-mails

The American Medical Association published the "Guidelines for Patient-Physician Electronic Mail" in 2004, since then other aspects have been added to the list [3]:

- Establish a turnaround time for reading new messages (time periods of the same part of the day).
- Inform patients of the appropriate use of e-mails (for what questions they should use it and who might see their e-mails).
- Do not use e-mail for medical emergencies.
- Ask patients to acknowledge that they read the reply for their message.
- Archive every e-mail.
- "Use a proper medical disclaimer in the bottom of each e-mail."
- Do not use e-mail for sensitive matters (e.g. HIV, mental health issues, etc.).
- E-mail communication is not a substitution for medical examination.
- Avoid anger, sarcasm, harsh criticism.

Privacy Concerns in Social Media

E-mail is only one form of communication with potential legal problems, but there are other platforms and resources in which private patient can accidentally be shared or inappropriate content can be published. Examples include:

- Sharing a case in a blog or in a Twitter message by mentioning identifiers described in the HIPAA act.
- Sharing medical images without hiding sensitive patient information.

- Publishing photos in social networking sites with alcohol or other inappropriate materials.
- Mixing personal and professional profiles and/or public opinions.
- Inappropriate prescribing and contact with patients online.
- Misinterpretation of credentials or clinical results.

In order to avoid such problems, certain aspects should always be kept in mind such as the protection of the privacy and confidentiality of patients, avoiding requests for online medical advice, acting with professionalism in every online activity and being aware of potential conflicts of interest, as well as that information posted online may be available to anyone and could be misconstrued [4].

Farris Timimi, M.D., medical director for the Mayo Clinic Center for Social Media, published a 12-word social media policy that might help medical professionals use social media in a secure way [5].

- Don't lie
- Don't pry (private health information should be discussed in online conversations)
- Don't cheat
- Can't delete
- Don't steal and give credit where it's due
- Don't reveal confidential information

Self-Test

1. What are some aspects of using e-mails as medical professionals?
   A turnaround time should be established, patients should be informed about the proper use of e-mails which should be archived.
2. What are the main concerns of using e-mails with patients?
   Inappropriate use for certain medical conditions; potential for increased physician workload; legal and privacy problems.

Key Points
- E-mail or electronic mail is a method of sending and receiving digital messages online.
- A medical disclaimer should be placed in the bottom of e-mails exchanged with patients.
- Different e-mail addresses should be used for personal and professional purposes.

References

1. Leong SL, et al. Enhancing doctor-patient communication using email: a pilot study. J Am Board Fam Med. 2005;18(3):180–8.
2. Neill RA, et al. The utility of electronic mail as a medium for patient-physician communication. Arch Fam Med. 1994;3(3):268–71.
3. Lewers DT. Guidelines for patient-physician electronic mail [monograph on the Internet]. Chicago: American Medical Association; 2000 [Cited 23 Dec 2004]. Available from: http://www.ama-assn.org/meetings/public/annual00/reports/bot/bot2a00.rtf. Accessed 28 Jan 2013.
4. 3 social media offenses to avoid. http://medicaleconomics.modernmedicine.com/news/3-social-media-offenses-avoid. Accessed 28 Jan 2013.
5. A 12-Word Social Media Policy. http://socialmedia.mayoclinic.org/2012/04/05/a-twelve-word-social-media-policy/. Accessed 28 Jan 2013.

Chapter 16
Social Bookmarking

Communication with patients and colleagues and being up-to-date in a field of interest can be time consuming and solutions saving time and effort are very much needed in the medical profession. It is also a common case that medical professionals have to work on different computers, laptops or mobile devices such as smartphones or tablets and synchronizing information is challenging.

Using different web browsers and web browser versions can lead to other accessibility problems. Social bookmarking provides a centralized online service enabling users to add, annotate, edit, and share bookmarks of web documents and sites [1, 2].

By assigning specific categories to these materials properly, finding the content in this user generated database is simple and accurate. The process is called tagging.

The main features of social bookmarking websites and services include:

- It saves the link or reference to the website, not the website itself.
- Metadata such as descriptions can be assigned to the websites.
- Websites can be tagged.
- Bookmark databases can be public or private only accessed by the user who created it.
- Ratings and comments are optional.

B. Meskó, *Social Media in Clinical Practice*,
DOI 10.1007/978-1-4471-4306-2_16,
© Springer-Verlag London 2013

TABLE 16.1   Examples of social bookmarking sites

Name	URL	Topics
CiteULike	http://www.citeulike.org/	Scholarly references
Mendeley	http://www.mendeley.com/	Academic social bookmarking
Del.icio.us	http://delicious.com	Non-specified
Digg	http://digg.com/	Non-specified
Diigo	http://www.diigo.com/	Non-specified
Reddit	http://www.reddit.com/	Non-specified
StumbleUpon	http://www.stumbleupon.com/	Non-specified

A typical user account shows the follower numbers as if our collection is public, users can follow that; number of links added, tags used, the websites that were added which can also be edited later on. Other platforms such as CiteULike or Connotea are specialized for scholarly references.

While URL shorteners create a database of the websites whose URL was shortened, there are services focusing only on social bookmarking (Table 16.1).

Self-Test

1. What are the most popular social bookmarking sites?
   Digg, Reddit, StumbleUpon and Mendeley.

Key Points
- Social bookmarking provides a centralized online service enabling users to add, annotate, edit, and share bookmarks of web documents and sites.
- By assigning specific categories to these materials properly, finding the content in this user generated database is simple and accurate.

References

1. Barton AJ. Social networking: social bookmarking tools [Abstract] Communicating Nursing Research Conference Proceedings. 2009
2. Angelova R, Marek L, Evangelos M, Pawel P. Investigating the properties of a social bookmarking and tagging network. IJDWM. 2010;6(1):1–19. Web. 28 Jan 2013. doi:10.4018/jdwm.2010090801.

Chapter 17
Conclusions

Social media has been clearly changing the way medicine is practiced and healthcare is delivered. The rising number of e-patients also initiated new movements in this area. Medical professionals of the twenty-first century must be able to meet the special needs of these patients and use digital technologies in their work and communication properly.

Web 2.0, Internet and social media represent the same concept: digital communication. While there is no difference among these expressions, social media can facilitate the workflow of medical professionals if used with strategy. Obviously, it cannot be a goal to transform all physicians into bloggers and Twitter users, but each physician should find the platforms, tools and solutions that can assist them in their workflow. Each case, each doctor's Internet use is different and requires specific skills.

New skills have to be acquired in the digital era:

- Being productive online is key.
- Building an online image for a medical professional or a practice requires planning, design and the thorough knowledge of social media.
- Dealing with e-mails with colleagues and patients in a proper and time-saving way.
- Knowing the privacy settings of different social media platforms by heart.
- Assessing the quality of websites, social media channels or even mobile apps. This is part of their responsibility now.

B. Meskó, *Social Media in Clinical Practice*,
DOI 10.1007/978-1-4471-4306-2_17,
© Springer-Verlag London 2013

- Prescribing information and online resources in an evidence based manner.
- Designing online campaigns for spreading the word about public health issues in the neighborhood or without geographical limits.
- Filtering the huge amount of information online.
- Building online professional community that could be used for crowdsourcing.

Patients looking for information and support online need to be educated how to use the online world; and it is the responsibility of medical professionals to contribute to this process. Building an online presence, communicating with patients or peers online, being up-to-date easily or finding the information they need must be common practices in medicine and healthcare. And as the same rules apply for real life as for the online world, similar approaches should be used and common sense should be in the focus.

There are some basic principles to keep in mind while using the Internet as a medical professional:

- Be transparent and clearly state who you are and what your intent is.
- Clarify your intent and make sure the rationale behind your activity is made clear.
- Select your audience as certain activities are only appropriate for specific audiences.
- Declare conflicts of interest.
- Follow the rules of social media platforms.
- The only way to fight against pseudoscience and medical quackery is to take control of publishing medical information on the web.
- By using social media platforms to ensure the quality of medical articles and blogs is appropriate, medical professionals can also build their online reputation.
- Platforms come and go, but the way a medical professional should communicate online and offline is constantly clear.

- If there is one place in the world where you cannot hide, this is the Internet. Always keep that in mind when posting any kind of content.
- Only post content online that is appropriate from every possible perspective.
- Social media is just a form of communication and it should be treated like that, no more, no less.

A summary of purposes social media platforms can be used for, although the sky is the limit:

- Building an online image for a medical professional or a practice.
- Keeping in touch with patients and colleagues worldwide.
- Organizing grand rounds, consultations and other group meetings.
- Keeping yourself up-to-date either in your field of interest or technology all together.
- Sharing thoughts, ideas, slideshows or cases.
- Helping your patients understand the proper use of the Internet as well as find quality medical information and resources online.
- Writing manuscripts collaboratively.

It is possible to use the constantly growing digital world in the practice of medicine efficiently with success in order to improve the care of patients and their relationship with medical professionals. But the only way to do so is the evidence-based, meaningful and strategic use of it. This handbook was a hopefully successful attempt at fulfilling this mission.

Links and Further Reading

1 Social Media Is Transforming Medicine and Healthcare

Google Chrome – http://www.google.com/chrome
Internet Explorer – http://windows.microsoft.com/en-US/internet-explorer/download-ie
Mozilla Firefox – http://www.mozilla.org
Safari – http://www.apple.com/safari
Twitter – http://twitter.com
Facebook – http://facebook.com
Youtube – http://youtube.com
Google+ – http://plus.google.com
Flickr – http://www.flickr.com
Twitter channel @Berci – https://twitter.com/Berci
Scienceroll medical blog – http://www.scienceroll.com
Webicina – http://www.webicina.com
HONcode – http://www.hon.ch/HONcode/Conduct.html

2 Using Medical Search Engines with a Special Focus on Google

AltaVista – http://www.altavista.com
Google – https://www.google.com
Bing – http://www.bing.com
Yahoo – http://www.yahoo.com
Ask – http://ask.com
AOL – http://www.aol.com

B. Meskó, *Social Media in Clinical Practice*,
DOI 10.1007/978-1-4471-4306-2,
© Springer-Verlag London 2013

DuckDuckGo – http://www.duckduckgo.com
A Google A Day – http://www.agoogleaday.com
Pubmed – http://www.pubmed.com
GoPubmed – http://www.gopubmed.org
BibliMed – http://www.biblimed.com
Pubget – http://pubget.com
Google Scholar – http://scholar.google.com
Wolfram Alpha – http://www.wolframalpha.com

3 Being Up-to-Date in Medicine

Feedly – http://www.feedly.com
My Yahoo – http://my.yahoo.com
Bloglines – http://www.bloglines.com
Feeddemon – http://www.feeddemon.com
Newsgator – http://netnewswireapp.com
Feed43 – http://www.feed43.com
PeRSSonalized Medicine – http://www.webicina.com/perssonalized
Medworm.com – http://www.medworm.com
Docphin – https://www.docphin.com
Google Alerts – http://www.google.com/alerts

4 Community Sites: Facebook, Google+ and Medical Social Networks

Facebook – http://www.facebook.com
Google+ – http://plus.google.com
LinkedIn – http://www.linkedin.com
FriendFeed – http://www.friendfeed.com
Ozmosis – http://www.ozmosis.com
Dxy – http://www.dxy.cn
Sermo – http://www.sermo.com
Doctors Hangout – http://www.doctorshangout.com
Doctors.net.uk – http://www.doctors.net.uk
Nature Network – http://network.nature.com
CMA – http://www.cma.ca
EchoJournal – http://www.echjournal.org
New Media Medicine – http://www.newmediamedicine.co
Doctrs – http://www.doctrs.com
Medcrowd – http://www.medcrowd.com
Esanum – http://www.esanum.com

5 The World of E-Patients

E-patients.net – http://www.e-patients.net
The Society for Participatory Medicine – http://participatorymedicine.org
The Journal of Participatory Medicine – http://www.jopm.org
Get Fit Slowly – http://getfitslowly.com
Dr Fitness & The Fat Guy – http://www.drfitnessandthefatguy.com
Fitness Wiki – http://fitness.wikia.com
Fitness Town – https://twitter.com/FitnessTown
Fitness Builder – https://www.fitnessbuilder.com
Vanity Health Club – http://www.youtube.com/user/VanityHealthClubs
Patientslikeme – http://www.patientslikeme.com
Inspire – http://www.inspire.com
MD Junction – http://www.mdjunction.com
Autism One – http://www.autismone.org
Cancer Forward – http://www.cancerforward.org
D Life – http://www.dlife.com
Baby Center – http://www.babycenter.com
Crohnology – http://crohnology.com
Maarten Lens-FitzGerald – http://maartensjourney.wordpress.com
Sixuntilme – http://www.sixuntilme.com
Lauren Parrott's Youtube channel – http://www.youtube.com/user/laurenvparrott
e-Patient Dave deBronkart – http://epatientdave.com
Kickbee on Twitter – http://kickbee.net

6 Establishing a Medical Blog

Photoblog – http://www.dianevarner.com
Personal blog – http://theinterpreterdiaries.com
Group blog – http://www.medgadget.com
Company blog – http://www.blogsouthwest.com
Videoblog – http://coachtvblog.com
Tematic blog – http://streetanatomy.com
Nurse blog – http://www.codeblog.com
Doctor blog – http://www.familymedicinerocks.com
Medical student blog – http://internal-optimist.blogspot.com
Medical lawyer blog – http://lawmedconsultant.com
Hospital manager blog – http://runningahospital.blogspot.com
Medical librarian blog – http://laikaspoetnik.wordpress.com
Patient blog – http://sixuntilme.com

Science of the Invisible – http://scienceoftheinvisible.blogspot.com/
NCBI ROFL – http://blogs.discovermagazine.com/discoblog
Wordpress.com – http://www.wordpress.com
Blogger – http://www.blogger.com
Typepad – http://www.typepad.com
Odiogo – http://www.odiogo.com
Google Analytics – https://www.google.com/analytics
Creative Commons – http://creativecommons.org

7 The Role of Twitter and Microblogging in Medicine

Twitter – http://www.twitter.com
Twitscoop – http://www.twitscoop.com
Twellow – http://www.twellow.com
WeFollow – http://www.wefollow.com
Bit.ly URL shortener – http://www.bit.ly
Ow.ly URL shortener – http://www.ow.ly
Paper.li – http://www.paper.li
Tweetdeck – http://www.tweetdeck.com
Organizations – https://twitter.com/WHOnews
Doctors – https://twitter.com/kevinmd
Medical journals – https://twitter.com/nejm
Hospitals – https://twitter.com/mayoclinic
Patients – https://twitter.com/sixuntilme
Friendfeed – http://www.friendfeed.com
Tumblr – http://www.tumblr.com

8 Collaboration Online

Skype – http://www.skype.com
Mikogo – http://www.mikogo.com
Oovoo – http://www.oovoo.com
FaceTalk – http://en.facetalk.nl
Facebook – http://www.facebook.com
Friendfeed – http://www.friendfeed.com
Grouptweet – http://www.grouptweet.com
Google Groups – http://groups.google.com
Wikispaces – http://www.wikispaces.com
Stixy – http://www.stixy.com
Mindmeister – http://www.mindmeister.com
Cacoo – http://www.cacoo.com
Dropbox – http://www.dropbox.com

Scribd – http://www.scribd.com
Gmail – http://www.gmail.com
Doodle – http://www.doodle.com
Google Docs – http://docs.google.com
Google Drive – http://drive.google.com
Zoho – http://www.zoho.com
Conceptboard – http://www.conceptboard.com

9 Wikipedia and Medical Wikis

MediaWiki – http://www.mediawiki.org
Wikispaces – http://www.wikispaces.com
Wikia – http://www.wikia.com
Askdrwiki – http://askdrwiki.com
Radiopaedia – http://radiopaedia.org
HLwiki – http://hlwiki.slais.ubc.ca
Ganfyd – http://www.ganfyd.org
FluWikie – http://www.fluwikie.com
WikiCancer – http://www.wikicancer.org
Clinfowiki – http://www.informatics-review.com
WikiKidney – http://wikikidney.org
Medpedia – http://www.medpedia.com
Wikipedia – http://en.wikipedia.org
Wiktionary – http://www.wiktionary.org
Wikibooks – http://www.wikibooks.org
Wikiversity – http://www.wikiversity.org
Wikinews – http://www.wikinews.org
Wikispecies – http://species.wikimedia.org
WikiMedia Commons – http://commons.wikimedia.org
Wikiquote – http://www.wikiquote.org
Wikisource – http://wikisource.org
WikiProject Medicine – http://en.wikipedia.org/wiki/Wikipedia:
    WikiProject_Medicine
Portal Medicine – http://en.wikipedia.org/wiki/Portal:Medicine
Assessment – http://en.wikipedia.org/wiki/Wikipedia:WikiProject_
    Medicine/Assessment
Collaboration of the month – http://en.wikipedia.org/wiki/Wikipedia:
    WikiProject_Medicine/Collaboration_of_the_Month

10 Organizing Medical Events
in Virtual Environments

Second Life – http://www.secondlife.com
Visuland – http://www.visuland.com

11 Medical Smartphone and Tablet Applications

Webicina – http://www.webicina.com
iMedicalApps – http://www.imedicalapps.com
Appolicious – http://www.appolicious.com/categories/26-health-fitness
AppBrain – http://www.appbrain.com/apps/highest-rated/medical/
AED4.eu – http://www.aed4.eu
Prognosis – http://www.prognosisapp.com
iDoc24 – http://idoc24.com

12 Use of Social Media by Hospitals and Medical Practices

Mayo Clinic – http://www.mayoclinic.com
Mayo Youtube channel – http://www.youtube.com/user/mayoclinic
Mayo Twitter channel – https://twitter.com/MayoClinic
Mayo Facebook page – http://www.facebook.com/MayoClinic
Mayo Blog – http://www.mayoclinic.org/blogs
Mayo Clinic Center for Social Media – http://socialmedia.mayoclinic.org
Mayo Connect – http://connect.mayoclinic.org

13 Medical Video and Podcast

Youtube – http://www.youtube.com
Fauquier ENT – http://www.youtube.com/user/fauquierent
HemOnc Today – http://www.youtube.com/user/HemOncToday
Society of General Internal Medicine – http://www.youtube.com/user/TheSGIM
European Society of Cardiology – http://www.youtube.com/user/escardiodotorg
Dr Jerry Gordon – http://www.youtube.com/user/DrJerryGordon
Clinical Neurology News – http://www.youtube.com/user/ClinNeurologyNews
Ustream – http://www.ustream.tv
Vimeo – http://vimeo.com
Justin.tv – http://www.justin.tv
Video, MD – http://www.videomd.com
eMedTV – http://www.emedtv.com
The Doctor's Channel – http://www.thedoctorschannel.com
OR Live – http://www.orlive.com
SciVee TV – http://www.scivee.tv

The Journal of the American Medical Association podcast – http://jama.
jamanetwork.com/multimedia.aspx#Weekly
The New England Journal of Medicine Weekly Summary podcast –
http://www.nejm.org/multimedia/audio-summary
The Medical University of South Carolina podcast – http://www.
muschealth.com/multimedia/Podcasts
Annals of Internal Medicine Podcast podcast – https://itunes.apple.com/
us/podcast/annals-internal-medicine-podcast/id259716343
Johns Hopkins Medicine News Roundup podcast – http://www.
hopkinsmedicine.org/news/audio/podcasts/
BlogTalkRadio – http://www.blogtalkradio.com
PodBean – http://www.podbean.com
PodOmatic – http://www.podomatic.com

14 Creating Presentations and Slideshows

Stockxpert – http://www.stockxpert.com
bigStockPhoto – http://www.bigstockphoto.com
Google Drive – https://drive.google.com
Dropbox – https://www.dropbox.com
Sliderocket – http://www.sliderocket.com
Prezi – http://www.prezi.com

16 Social Bookmarking

CiteULike – http://www.citeulike.org
Mendeley – http://www.mendeley.com
Delicious – http://delicious.com
Digg – http://digg.com
Diigo – http://www.diigo.com
Reddit – http://www.reddit.com
StumbleUpon – http://www.stumbleupon.com

Index

B. Meskó, *Social Media in Clinical Practice*,
DOI 10.1007/978-1-4471-4306-2,
© Springer-Verlag London 2013

Lightning Source UK Ltd.
Milton Keynes UK
UKOW05f0330051013

218524UK00018B/901/P